# ARE YOU KI[DDING ME?]

*Alternative recipes fo[r] dairy-free and [gluten-free]*

**All natural, healthy and organic recipes that taste good!**

MW00427266

**C. A. Torella, Healthy Living Advocate**

Dedicated to my parents Dorothy and Bob.
For your never-ending support, love and
encouragement.

With great thanks to my Dad who taught
me so many things and showed me that love
of food and passion for cooking would always
have great rewards.

Disclaimer:
The recipes and opinions expressed in this book are those of the author. Any information contained reflects the author's experiences and is not intended in any way to take the place of medical advice from a health care professional. Some recipes may contain some ingredients that may not be suitable for all diets. Always consult a medical health care professional for anything in question.

# TIPS

### Cheese/cheese substitute
Several non-dairy cheese options are available at many supermarkets, health food and specialty stores. Goat or sheep cheese is often easier to digest if you're sensitive. Nutritional yeast is an excellent substitute for vegetarian, gluten-free, salt-free, sugar-free diets, and provides a significant amount of B vitamins. It is versatile enough to use in any recipe.

### Cinnamon
Organic cinnamon is an excellent metabolism booster and great flavour enhancer for an endless list of dishes. Add it to your favorite latte, smoothie, salad, stir fry, rice, sauce, salad dressing, etc.

### Egg substitute
1 tbsp. of ground flax seed with 3 tbsp. of water is equivalent to 1 whole egg. Stir together and let sit for approximately 3 minutes before adding to a recipe.

### Flours that are gluten and wheat-free
Amaranth, arrowroot, brown rice, buckwheat, chia, chickpea, coconut, hemp, millet, potato, quinoa, sorghum, tapioca and white rice flour. When substituting flours, the best results are achieved by using two or three together instead of just one type of flour. For example; if a recipe calls for 1 cup of all-purpose flour; substitute for 1/2 cup of chickpea flour and 2/3 cup of brown rice flour.

### Food wash
Wash all fruits and vegetables with a biodegradable, anti-bacterial food wash.

### Grains
Grains that contain gluten include; wheat, barley, kamut, oat, rye, spelt. Non-glutinous products include; amaranth, buckwheat, chickpea, coconut, flaxseed, millet, potato, quinoa, soy, tapioca.

## Himalayan pink sea salt

It is said to be the purest form of sea salt. Himalayan salts are mineral packed crystals which formed naturally within the earth include: magnesium, calcium, potassium, bicarbonate, bromide and borate. These minerals can create an electrolyte balance, increase hydration, balance pH and help to reduce acid reflux, prevent muscle cramping, strengthen bones, aid in proper metabolism function, lower blood pressure, help intestines absorb nutrients and improve circulation.

## Kale

Several types of kale are available; likely the most common is curly, tuscan/black and purple. If you cannot find kale you could substitute for swiss chard or spinach.

## Legumes

Also known as beans, peas and lentils are a high-fiber, low-fat source of protein, loaded with vitamins and also extremely versatile. They are available dried or canned and both types are equally nutritious and handy to have in the cupboard. They make a great substitute for meat, poultry or fish. Legumes are also packed with calcium, iron, folic acid, zinc, potassium, magnesium and B vitamins.

## Milk alternatives

Almond, cashew, coconut, hemp, rice, soy; all come in various flavours as well as low fat and unsweetened. Each has a different taste and all are great dairy-free options.

## Nut or seed butters

Almond, cashew, coconut, macadamia nut, peanut, pistachio, pumpkin seed, sesame seed, soy nut, sunflower seed, walnut. Many of these are available in a grocery or health food store, or why not make your own. I prefer to start with raw nuts and seeds as they offer more nutritional value than roasted.

## Nutritional yeast

An excellent substitute for cheese because of its taste. Don't let the name fool you; nutritional yeast flakes may be one of the best additions to your diet. It provides a wealth of vitamins, minerals and protein that almost anyone from Paleo to vegan can enjoy. Nutritional yeast is packed with B-vitamins, folic acid, selenium, zinc, and protein. It's low in fat, gluten-free and contains no added sugars or preservatives. It is a great addition to any diet!

## Organics

Choose organic whenever possible as it is free of pesticides, chemicals, additives and preservatives. When unavailable be careful with porous fruits as the pesticides penetrate right into the fruit and washing or scrubbing cannot remove them completely. Also, if organic is not handy then local is better than a large chain store.

## Protein sources

Some excellent sources of protein are: salmon, halibut, octopus, anchovies, tuna, lean beef, chicken, turkey, beans, lentils, peanuts, almonds, tofu, quinoa, yogurt, eggs, cottage cheese.

## Quinoa

It is pronounced "Keen-wah" and contains more protein than any other grain; is a good source of dietary fiber, high in magnesium, potassium and iron. It is also a good source of phosphorous, calcium, vitamin E and several B vitamins which can be used instead of pasta, rice or couscous.

Quinoa flakes or brown rice flakes look similar to oatmeal flakes and can often be found in a bulk store, health food or specialty store, and they are a great addition to homemade granola.

## Restaurant eating

Be cautious of items like salad dressing, condiments and sauces that may not be made from scratch as these items are usually full of sugar and sodium as well as preservatives, additives and dyes. Depending on allergies or food restrictions a good alternative is to request separate oil and vinegar to replace a dressing or lemon or lime wedges. Don't be afraid to ask to see the label or ingredient list of any item in question. If you are unfamiliar with the restaurant, check their website or call to get menu items and if unsure of any good choices, I will often eat before I go and then just order a small item to stay part of the social environment and I also frequently have a source of protein or a snack with me just in case.

## Shopping

A local farmers market with organics will often have the freshest selections as they are the closest so this is my preference, but even non-organic produce at the market will be a better alternative to supermarket produce that comes from another country. Home delivery of organics may be an option in your community which is very convenient for busy families. Many bulk stores carry a wide selection of organic dry goods, nuts, cereals and some canned goods at a lower cost than other stores. Specialty stores and health stores will carry a more extensive selection of organics and all-natural, chemical-free items and often you can place special orders for unique or hard to find items; don't be afraid to ask for assistance. Superstores will usually have a wide selection of frozen organics throughout the year when fresh is difficult to find, and they will also carry a large variety of non-dairy options to choose from.

## Soaking and sprouting nuts and seeds

Soak any raw nuts in water for a few hours or overnight to increase the nutritional value, increase the protein availability, increase the fiber content and to make them easier to digest. Almonds, cashews, hazelnuts, macadamias, pecans, pistachios and walnuts can all be soaked. These nuts may not actually sprout. The following are some excellent beans, legumes and seeds to sprout as well. Be sure these are raw, uncooked: Adzuki beans, black beans, chickpeas, kidney beans, lentils, mung beans, navy beans, peas and quinoa. Check a proper soaking/sprouting chart for further instructions and best results.

## Sugar (white) alternatives

Organic cane sugar, coconut sugar, organic raw honey, organic maple syrup, stevia, molasses, xylitol. All of these options are a better choice than refined, processed (white) sugar.

## Tomatoes

To prevent flavor loss in your tomatoes, don't put them in the fridge! If they are starting to get soft, they can be frozen for future cooking purposes instead of discarding them. Simply wash and freeze whole in airtight freezer bags. Take straight from the freezer and rinse under hot water for a minute to remove skin. Chopping is very easy when tomatoes are still frozen but they retain water so adjust recipes accordingly or drain thoroughly.

## Travelling with allergies and food restrictions

It can be very challenging and stressful to think of travelling with food allergies so the best advice is to plan ahead. Whether going to another city or to another country you can do some research and planning. Prepare snacks for the car or to pack in your suitcase. A good source of protein is nuts, seeds, homemade energy mix, some organic cereals, milk alternatives in a carton (not refrigerated); these all travel well. You can research the food that is local to where you'll be and also research restaurants in the areas you're visiting to read the menu ahead of time and plan for what you can have. Often, I will find a local store that I can purchase items in that I know are safe for me and then I may also eat something before or after going to a restaurant so that I have had sufficient protein and nutrients.

# BREAKFAST AND BRUNCH

# Dairy-free Pancakes

1/3 cup brown rice four
1/3 cup amaranth flour
2 tsp. gluten-free baking powder
Pinch of Himalayan pink sea salt, fine ground
1 egg equivalent*
3/4 cup almond milk (or other if preferred)
2 tsp. organic extra virgin olive oil, grapeseed oil or avocado oil
2 tsp. organic liquid honey
1 cup organic berries, washed

*1 egg equivalent: 1 tbsp. ground flax seed mixed with 3 tbsp. of water
and let stand for 2 minutes then mix together

Blend flours, baking powder and sea salt together in a bowl.
Whisk the egg equivalent with the almond milk and olive oil, then
pour into the dry ingredients and blend together roughly with
a fork. Add the liquid honey and blend until smooth. Heat a
non-stick pan with a few drops of olive oil. Drop batter from a
large spoon and create small medallion size pancakes or larger
if preferred. When edges start to thicken and curl and bottom is
browning, flip over carefully. New batches may require more drops
of oil to prevent sticking and burning. Serve with fresh berries and
top with organic maple syrup.

*Be sure to check the beginning of the book in the TIPS section for many helpful
hints, alternatives, substitutes or suggestions that could save time and energy!*

# Energy Snack

1 cup organic raw almonds
1 cup organic raisins
1/2 cup organic raw cashews (whole or pieces)
1/2 cup organic raw sunflower seeds
1/2 cup dairy-free semi-sweet chocolate chips
1/2 cup goji berries
1/4 cup hemp seeds

Mix all together and keep in an airtight container. Scoop into zip lock baggies to take with you anytime you want an energy boost.

Optional: add 1 tsp. organic cayenne pepper, organic cinnamon or dried organic ginger to change the flavour and give a little kick.

*Be sure to check the beginning of the book in the TIPS section for many helpful hints, alternatives, substitutes or suggestions that could save time and energy!*

# Quick Breakfast Cereal or Anytime Trail Mix

1/3 cup organic brown rice flakes
1/3 cup organic walnuts
1 – 2 tbsp. organic apricots, chopped
1/3 cup raw organic pumpkin seeds
1/4 cup organic currants or raisins
1/4 cup organic coconut flakes
Almond milk (optional)

Mix all together and enjoy with milk for breakfast or just have it dry anytime as a healthy energy boosting snack. For a sweet treat add 1/3 cup organic unsweetened carob or dairy-free chocolate chips.

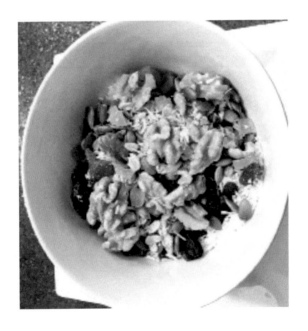

*Be sure to check the beginning of the book in the TIPS section for many helpful hints, alternatives, substitutes or suggestions that could save time and energy!*

## Just Like Chocolate for Breakfast

1/3 cup organic brown rice flakes
1 cup water
1 tbsp. unsweetened carob or dairy-free chocolate chips
1/4 cup chopped walnuts and finely chopped currants (if desired)
1 tbsp. organic pure maple syrup

Bring water and brown rice flakes to a boil for 1 minute, add currants and walnuts and cook for 2 minutes. Add carob chips and remove from heat. Stir just enough to mix through then spoon into serving bowl. Top with pure maple syrup.

For a festive variation; use 1/2 cup whole organic cranberries instead of nuts and currants.

*Be sure to check the beginning of the book in the TIPS section for many helpful hints, alternatives, substitutes or suggestions that could save time and energy!*

# Hot Creamy Breakfast Cereal

1/3 cup organic quinoa flakes or brown rice flakes
1/2 cup of your favorite organic berries
1 tbsp. pure or organic maple syrup
1/4 cup walnuts, chopped (optional)
1 tsp. organic cinnamon (optional)
Almond milk (optional)

Add flakes to 1 cup of boiling water, return to a boil and cook for 2 minutes, stirring frequently. Remove from heat, add berries and blend just enough to mix. Spoon into serving bowl, pour maple syrup over top and serve. I find this creamy as is but if you want it creamier add some of your favorite milk. Add chopped walnuts if desired.
Makes one serving; double or triple for more.

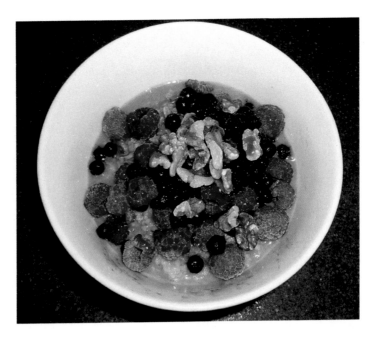

*Be sure to check the beginning of the book in the TIPS section for many helpful hints, alternatives, substitutes or suggestions that could save time and energy!*

# Scrambled Egg White Breakfast Wrap

Sprouted wrap, gluten-free or brown rice wrap
1/4-1/2 cup organic egg whites only
1/3 cup goat marble cheese, grated, dairy-free cheese substitute or nutritional yeast
1/3 cup slivered sweet pepper (red, yellow or orange)
Extra virgin olive oil, grapeseed oil or avocado oil
Himalayan pink sea salt and pepper to taste

Whip egg whites. Pour a few drops of the oil in a pan and heat. Whip the eggs as they are poured into the pan. Add the peppers and scramble until cooked. Spread over toasted wrap. Add cheese, sea salt and roll it up.

Optional: substitute cheese with organic salsa.

Heating the pan with the oil before adding the food will prevent the oil from being absorbed into the food.

*Be sure to check the beginning of the book in the TIPS section for many helpful hints, alternatives, substitutes or suggestions that could save time and energy!*

# Nut/Seed Butter Breakfast Wrap

Sprouted wrap, gluten-free or brown rice wrap
Organic pumpkin seed butter
1/4-1/2 cup grated goat's milk mozzarella or dairy-free cheese substitute

Spread pumpkin butter all over the wrap and add cheese on top.
Toast in toaster oven or conventional oven until crispy and cheese
is melting. Roll up and enjoy!

Optional: substitute cheese with organic honey.
Optional: substitute pumpkin seed butter with organic almond or
nut-free butter.

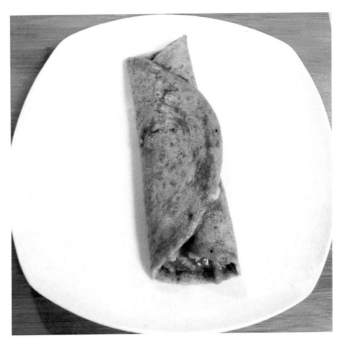

*Be sure to check the beginning of the book in the TIPS section for many helpful
hints, alternatives, substitutes or suggestions that could save time and energy!*

# Kale Omelette

3 whole eggs or 1/2 cup organic egg whites
2-3 leaves organic kale, chopped small and stem removed
1/4 cup organic red onion, chopped
2 tbsp. organic hot salsa
1-2 tsp. organic extra virgin olive oil, grapeseed oil or avocado oil
Himalayan pink sea salt and pepper to taste


Wash kale leaves. Heat oil in an omelette pan; add onion and sauté on med heat until tender. Add chopped kale and cook for about 5 minutes. Pour in whipped eggs/whites, cover and reduce heat to med-low, cooking until egg is done around the edges and browning on the bottom; carefully flip over. Spoon salsa on top and cover again for approx 2-3 minutes until all egg is cooked.

Optional: substitute hot salsa for mild or medium, if preferred.

*Be sure to check the beginning of the book in the TIPS section for many helpful hints, alternatives, substitutes or suggestions that could save time and energy!*

# Quinoa Breakfast Bites

1/2 cup quinoa
1 1/2 cup zucchini, grated
1/3 cup red pepper, chopped small
1/4 cup spinach, chopped small
2 brown free-run eggs (or egg substitute)
4 egg whites or 1/2 cup
1/2 cup goat cheddar, goat marble or dairy-free cheese substitute
1/2 tsp. organic hot sauce
Himalayan pink sea salt and pepper

Cook the quinoa per the package instructions. Preheat the oven to 350°. Whisk the eggs and egg whites together in a large bowl and then add all remaining ingredients to combine together. Spray a 12 section muffin tin with cooking spray or use paper liners. Pour the mixture evenly into the section. Bake for approximately 30 minutes or until golden and a toothpick inserted in the center comes out clean.

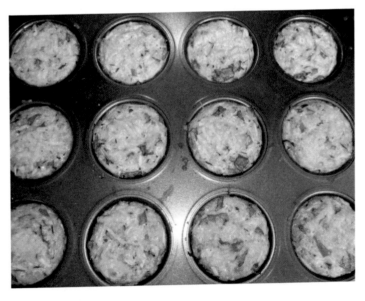

*Be sure to check the beginning of the book in the TIPS section for many helpful hints, alternatives, substitutes or suggestions that could save time and energy!*

# Italian Omelette

3 whole eggs or 1/2 cup organic egg whites
1 1/4cup organic zucchini, grated
1/3 cup organic red pepper, chopped
1/4 cup fresh organic basil, chopped
1 tbsp. organic hot sauce
2 tsp. extra virgin olive oil, grapeseed oil or avocado oil
Himalayan pink sea salt and pepper to taste

Wash vegetables. On medium heat, sauté the zucchini and peppers in oil until tender. Add hot sauce, salt and pepper to eggs and beat together. Pour eggs into pan and cover with a lid, cooking approximately 5 minutes until egg is firming up. Flip over, cover again and reduce heat to low, continuing to cook for a few minutes until all egg is cooked through.

Serve with whole grain sprouted muffin or gluten free toast.

*Be sure to check the beginning of the book in the TIPS section for many helpful hints, alternatives, substitutes or suggestions that could save time and energy!*

# Egg White Omelette with Spinach and Asparagus

1 cup organic egg whites
1 cup packed organic spinach, chopped
4 spears organic asparagus, chopped small
2 tsp. organic extra virgin olive oil, grapeseed oil or avocado oil
Himalayan pink sea salt and pepper to taste

Wash the vegetables and dry before chopping. Heat the pan with oil. Beat the egg whites with a fork until bubbles form and pour into the pan. Add the spinach and asparagus and cook covered on med heat until egg is white and browning on the bottom. Flip over and grind some fresh sea salt and pepper to taste. Reduce heat to simmer and cover with lid. Cook until browning on bottom. Fold half over and flip onto plate.

Heating the pan with the oil before adding the food will prevent the oil from being absorbed into the food.

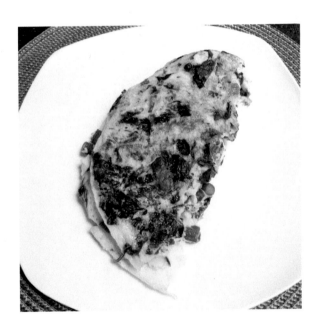

*Be sure to check the beginning of the book in the TIPS section for many helpful hints, alternatives, substitutes or suggestions that could save time and energy!*

## Almond Power Smoothie

1 cup organic unsweetened almond milk
2 tbsp. raw nut butter (almond, pumpkin, cashew)
2 tsp. fresh ground flax seed
1/2 ripe avocado
1 kale leaf, chopped small
A dash of organic cinnamon
1 scoop or 1 serving of whole food-based protein powder

Pour milk first into a Vitamix or high-powered blender. Add all remaining ingredients and blend until smooth. Feel free to add more milk or filtered water to thin it down if you feel it's too thick.

*Be sure to check the beginning of the book in the TIPS section for many helpful hints, alternatives, substitutes or suggestions that could save time and energy!*

# Antioxidant Smoothie

1 cup organic unsweetened almond milk
1/3 cup organic blueberries
1/3 cup organic raspberries
1/3 cup organic blackberries
1 tbsp. chia seeds
1 scoop or 1 serving of whole food-based protein powder

Pour milk first into a Vitamix or high-powered blender. Add all remaining ingredients and blend until smooth. Feel free to add more milk or filtered water to thin it down if you feel it's too thick.

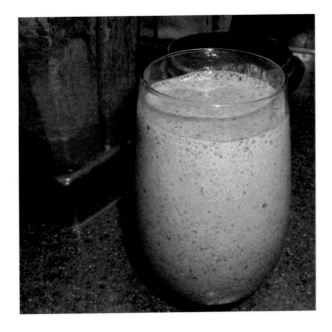

*Be sure to check the beginning of the book in the TIPS section for many helpful hints, alternatives, substitutes or suggestions that could save time and energy!*

## Blueberry Breakfast Smoothie

1 cup almond milk
1 cup frozen blueberries
1/2 ripe avocado or 1/2 ripe banana, cut up
1tbsp. ground flax seed
1 tsp. maca powder
1 tsp. chia seeds
1 tsp. organic cinnamon
1 scoop or 1 serving of whole food-based protein powder

Pour milk first into a Vitamix or high-powered blender then add all remaining ingredients and blend until smooth.

Optional: substitute almond for coconut, cashew, hemp or rice milk.

*Be sure to check the beginning of the book in the TIPS section for many helpful hints, alternatives, substitutes or suggestions that could save time and energy!*

# Detox Smoothie

1 cup all-natural coconut water
1 cup frozen or fresh mango
1/2 ripe avocado
1/2 cup cilantro
3/4 cup greens (spinach, lettuce, kale)
1 tsp. grated fresh ginger
1 organic lemon, juice squeezed
2 tsp. raw unpasteurized honey
1 tbsp. shredded organic unsweetened coconut
Dash of organic cinnamon (optional)

Pour coconut water first into a Vitamix or high-powered blender then add all remaining ingredients and blend until smooth.

Optional: substitute lime for lemon if preferred.
Optional: if cilantro is not to your liking you can add more greens.

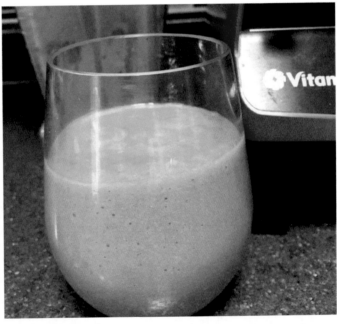

*Be sure to check the beginning of the book in the TIPS section for many helpful hints, alternatives, substitutes or suggestions that could save time and energy!*

# Green Smoothie

1 cup organic unsweetened coconut milk
1/3 cup organic blueberries
1/3 cup organic raspberries
1 tsp. liquid chlorophyll
1 tbsp. greens powder
1 tsp. maca powder
1 tsp. chia seeds
A dash of organic cinnamon
1 scoop (1/4 cup) organic plant-based protein powder

Pour milk first into a Vitamix or high-powered blender. Add all remaining ingredients and blend until smooth. Feel free to add more milk or filtered water to thin it down if you feel it's too thick.

*Be sure to check the beginning of the book in the TIPS section for many helpful hints, alternatives, substitutes or suggestions that could save time and energy!*

# Raspberry and Mango Smoothie

1 1/2 cup unsweetened raw cashew milk
1 cup frozen organic raspberries
1/2 cup frozen mango
1 tsp. ground flax seed
1 scoop (1/4 cup) organic plant-based protein powder
1 tsp. maca powder

*Raw cashew milk, recipe pg. 28*

Pour milk first into a Vitamix or high-powered blender. Add all remaining ingredients and blend until smooth. Feel free to add more milk or filtered water to thin it down if you feel it's too thick.

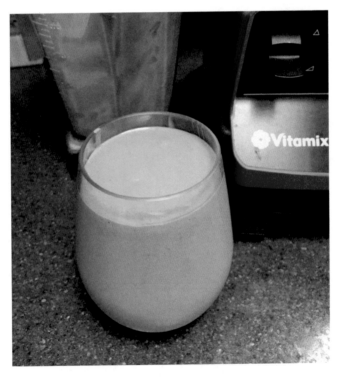

*Be sure to check the beginning of the book in the TIPS section for many helpful hints, alternatives, substitutes or suggestions that could save time and energy!*

# Raw Almond Milk

1 cup raw almonds (organic preferred)
8 cups filtered water, separated

Soak almonds in 4 cups filtered water for 8 hours or overnight. Drain and discard water. Place almonds in a 2L capacity Vitamix or high-powered blender. Add 4 cups of fresh filtered water. Turn on blender and slowly increase the speed to 10 and then switch to high for 45-50 seconds. I like to use this milk for smoothies so I keep the nut-meal intact and simply pour it into mason jars and store in the fridge. If desired, you can use a milk bag to squeeze the milk into a large bowl and then pour into mason jars and store in the fridge. Always give a good shake to the milk before using and it's best to use it up in 4-5 days.
The nut-meal can be saved, spread on a cookie sheet and dried in the oven at 175° for approx 2 hours. This can be used in cereal, smoothies, soups, salads, etc.

Optional: sweeten if preferred, by adding any one of the following for a variety of flavours:
1 tsp. organic vanilla extract or organic coconut extract
1 tbsp. organic maple syrup
4 pitted dates
(Return to blender with milk to mix thoroughly together)

*Be sure to check the beginning of the book in the TIPS section for many helpful hints, alternatives, substitutes or suggestions that could save time and energy!*

## Raw Cashew Milk

1 cup raw cashews (organic preferred)
8 cups filtered water, separated

Soak cashews in 4 cups filtered water for 8 hours or overnight. Drain and discard water. Place cashews in a 2L capacity Vitamix or high-powered blender. Add 4 cups of fresh filtered water. Turn on blender and slowly increase the speed to 10 and then switch to high for 45-50 seconds. There is no need to filter the cashews as they don't produce the same nut-meal as almonds. Simply pour into mason jars and keep in the fridge. Always give a good shake to the milk before using and it's best to use it up in 4-5 days.

Optional: sweeten if preferred, by adding any one of the following for a variety of flavours:
1 tsp. organic vanilla or organic coconut extract
1 tbsp. organic maple syrup
4 pitted dates
(Return to blender with milk to mix thoroughly together)

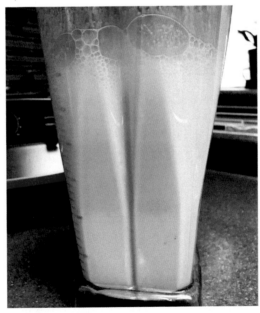

*Be sure to check the beginning of the book in the TIPS section for many helpful hints, alternatives, substitutes or suggestions that could save time and energy!*

# SNACKS, LUNCHES AND SALADS

## Anytime Dip for Veggies or Crackers

1/2 cup hummus (roasted red pepper, onion, garlic or plain)
1/2 cup organic medium salsa

Mix together in a bowl until well blended and serve with your
favourite selection of sliced veggies, rice crackers, tortilla chips or
all of the above.

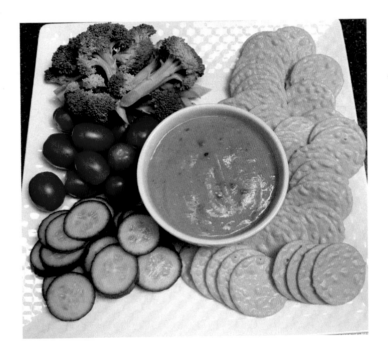

*Be sure to check the beginning of the book in the TIPS section for many helpful
hints, alternatives, substitutes or suggestions that could save time and energy!*

## Crostini Made Easy

2 slices of your favourite gluten-free bread or sliced bun
1–2 tbsp. olive oil
1/4 cup sliced kalamato olives
Organic balsamic glaze
Himalayan pink sea salt and pepper to taste

Cut bread slices (or bun) in half diagonally. Brush lightly with olive oil on one side. Grill in oven or BBQ for a few minutes, until lightly browned. Add sliced olives, a sprinkle of salt and pepper and then drizzle balsamic glaze over top and serve.

*Be sure to check the beginning of the book in the TIPS section for many helpful hints, alternatives, substitutes or suggestions that could save time and energy!*

## Veggie Pizza

1/2 cup broccoli, chopped
1/2 cup kale, chopped
1/2 cup red, yellow or orange pepper, chopped thin
1/4 cup onion, chopped fine
1/2 cup marinara sauce
3/4 cup grated goat mozzarella cheese, dairy-free cheese substitute or nutritional yeast
Substitute any vegetable above if preferred.

Spread sauce all over pizza crust, top with vegetables evenly distributed. Spread grated cheese or cheese substitute on top. Place a sheet of parchment paper on a baking sheet and bake the pizza at 375° for 15-20 minutes, or desired browning.

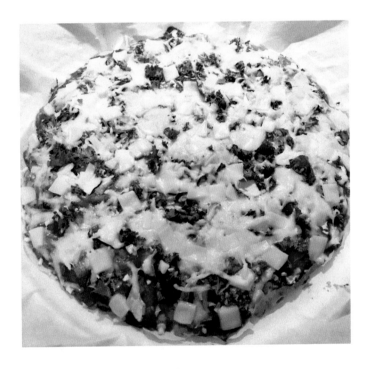

*Be sure to check the beginning of the book in the TIPS section for many helpful hints, alternatives, substitutes or suggestions that could save time and energy!*

# Chickpea Pizza Crust

2 cups chickpea flour
1 cup water
2 tbsp. olive oil
1/4 tsp. Himalayan pink sea salt
1–2 tsp. dried basil
1–2 tsp. dried oregano

Mix all ingredients in a bowl with a fork and blend until smooth. Preheat oven to 375°. Line a 13" round pizza pan with parchment paper and pour the batter mixture on the paper in a circular motion. Use the back of a spoon and continue to smooth out to all edged and evenly distribute for the same thickness. Bake for 18-20 minutes until lightly browning. Remove from heat and top with your favourite toppings.

*Be sure to check the beginning of the book in the TIPS section for many helpful hints, alternatives, substitutes or suggestions that could save time and energy!*

## Avocado, Tuna and Celery

1 organic avocado, soft
1 can organic tuna packed in water
2 stalks organic celery, chopped
1 tbsp. organic soy or non-diary mayonnaise substitute
1 tbsp. fresh lemon juice
Himalayan pink sea salt and pepper to taste

Cut avocado in half and scoop out into mixing bowl. Drain
the tuna, flake and add to the avocado. Add soy or non-diary
mayonnaise and celery, lemon juice, sea salt and pepper and mix
all together.

Serve on: your favorite rice crackers, wraps, or muffins; try toasting
them for another variation.

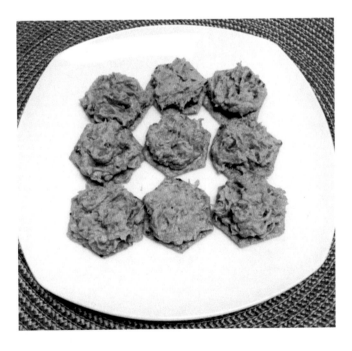

*Be sure to check the beginning of the book in the TIPS section for many helpful
hints, alternatives, substitutes or suggestions that could save time and energy!*

## Mexican Tortilla Pizza

Brown rice tortillas or any gluten-free wrap of your choice
Organic medium salsa
Organic red onion, thinly sliced
Soft goat's milk cheese, grated goat mozzarella cheese, dairy-free
cheese substitute or nutritional yeast

Lightly toast the tortillas for a few minutes. Place on a pizza pan,
spoon a thin layer of salsa evenly all over. Spread some thinly
sliced onion and top with cheese. Bake in 350° oven for 10-15
minutes until cheese is melted.

Optional: turn the heat up or down but substituting medium for
hot or mild salsa.

*Be sure to check the beginning of the book in the TIPS section for many helpful
hints, alternatives, substitutes or suggestions that could save time and energy!*

# Easy Bean Dip

1 can organic bean – your choice (kidney, black, pinto)
1 1/3 cup organic salsa – mild or medium

Rinse and drain the beans then transfer to a medium size bowl. With the back of a fork, mash the beans until pretty smooth. Add the salsa and stir together, continuing to mash with the fork until well blended.

Serve with your favorite crackers, vegetable slices or as a nice side dish to eggs.

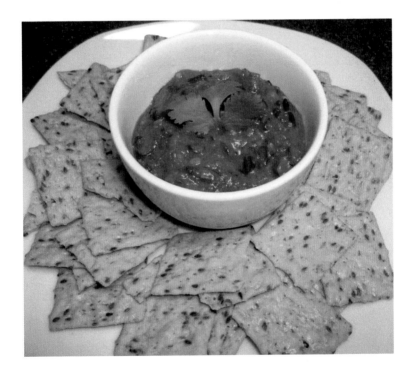

*Be sure to check the beginning of the book in the TIPS section for many helpful hints, alternatives, substitutes or suggestions that could save time and energy!*

## Garlic Paste for Toast

2-3 garlic cloves
1/3–1/2 cup coconut oil, butter or margarine

Optional: few drops of lemon juice
Optional: 1/2 tsp. chopped parsley, cilantro or basil
Optional: 1/4 cup of shredded vegan cheese, cheddar, goat marble or
your preferred choice

Add the coconut oil, butter or margarine to a bowl and blend
with the back of a spoon until smooth. Peel outer skin from garlic
cloves, squeeze the garlic through a press or mash into a pulp.
Add this, including any garlic juice to the oil and mix thoroughly.

Spread lightly on your favourite bread, bun or bagel and place on
a piece of parchment paper. Toast under the broiler on low until
browning and or cheese is bubbling.

Serve on: gluten-free bagel, bun or bread, pumpernickel or rye.

*Be sure to check the beginning of the book in the TIPS section for many helpful
hints, alternatives, substitutes or suggestions that could save time and energy!*

# Tortilla Nachos with Salsa

2 Brown rice or gluten-free thin tortillas
1 cup organic salsa – hot, med or mild
1 tsp. organic extra virgin olive oil, grapeseed oil or avocado oil

Lightly brush the tortillas with the oil of your choice. Place tortillas right on the oven rack and gently brown and crisp for approximately 10 – 15 minutes at 300°. Turn if necessary. Let cool on a drying rack before cutting. Cut into triangles and serve with salsa.

Optional: add 1 tbsp. soft goat, dairy-free cheese substitute or nutritional yeast to the salsa for a creamy variation and heat, if desired.

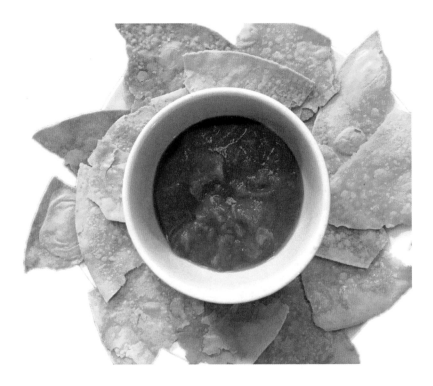

*Be sure to check the beginning of the book in the TIPS section for many helpful hints, alternatives, substitutes or suggestions that could save time and energy!*

## Cucumber with Nut Butter

1 cup english cucumber, sliced
1/2 cup organic almond, pumpkin or soy nut butter
Gluten-free, wheat-free crackers

Slice cucumber into rounds. Spread the butter of our choice on the cucumber slices. Place on your favorite cracker or a variety of options and serve.

*Be sure to check the beginning of the book in the TIPS section for many helpful hints, alternatives, substitutes or suggestions that could save time and energy!*

# Mixed Greens with Roasted Turkey

1 1/2 cup organic mixed greens
1/4 cup organic red onion, chopped fine
1 1/2 cups roasted turkey, diced
1/2 cup organic cucumber, sliced thin
1/2 cup organic grape tomatoes
Himalayan pink sea salt and pepper to taste
Optional: add 2 tbsp. dried cranberries

*Serve with Balsamic Vinaigrette, pg. 66*

Wash all greens and spin to dry. Wash vegetables. Tear greens into bite size pieces and put in med sized bowl. Add cucumber, tomatoes, onion and turkey and toss well. Pour vinegar first then oil and mix throughout. Top with dried cranberries if (desired) and fresh ground sea salt and pepper.

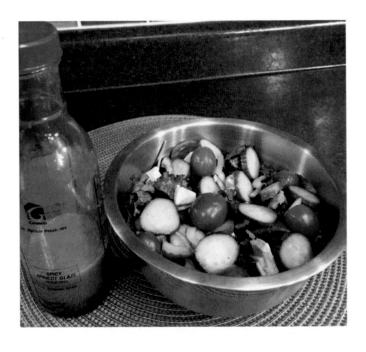

*Be sure to check the beginning of the book in the TIPS section for many helpful hints, alternatives, substitutes or suggestions that could save time and energy!*

## *Afternoon Energy Snack*

1–2 pieces of fresh fruit – apple, pear, watermelon, honeydew
1/4 cup raw almond butter, organic pumpkin seed butter or nut-free butter

Cut the fruit in slices and discard any seeds or core.
(If packing your snack for later simply drizzle a little lemon juice
in the tight-sealing container or bag with the fruit to keep it from
browning)
Dip or spread the butter on your fruit and enjoy.

*Be sure to check the beginning of the book in the TIPS section for many helpful*
*hints, alternatives, substitutes or suggestions that could save time and energy!*

# Arugula and Kale Salad

1 1/2 cup arugula
2 leaves curly kale
1/4 cup red onion
1/2 cup grape tomatoes
1/3 cup broccoli stems, peeled and slivered
1/2 cup organic english cucumber, sliced
1/4 cup walnuts, cut in half
1 tbsp. roasted chick peas (optional)

*Serve with Mustard Dressing, pg. 73*
Wash all vegetables. Remove stem from kale if desired. Tear kale
and arugula in smaller pieces, add to bowl. Chop onion finely.
Sliver the broccoli and cucumber. Add all ingredients to the bowl,
pour some mustard dressing over and toss gently to mix together.

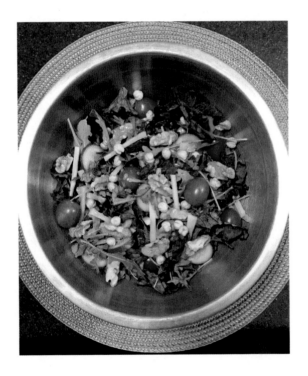

*Be sure to check the beginning of the book in the TIPS section for many helpful
hints, alternatives, substitutes or suggestions that could save time and energy!*

## Salmon Wrap

Gluten-free wrap of your choice
1 cooked salmon fillet, flaked
Organic tomatoes, diced
Organic asparagus spears, shredded
Organic mustard
Organic soy mayonnaise or dairy-free mayonnaise substitute


Wash vegetables. Dice tomato, shred asparagus enough for the number of wraps desired. Warm the fish slightly so that it flakes easily. Warm the tortilla shell when you are all ready to mix your wrap. Place the warmed wrap on a sheet of wax paper, spread with mustard and mayonnaise then add the fish and top with shredded asparagus and tomatoes. Roll up folding in the bottom to keep contents intact.

*Be sure to check the beginning of the book in the TIPS section for many helpful hints, alternatives, substitutes or suggestions that could save time and energy!*

# Avocado, Cucumber and Tomato Salad

1/2 avocado sliced
1 organic mini cucumber or 1/2 cup english cucumber, sliced
4–6 organic cherry or grape tomatoes, sliced in half
1 tbsp. organic lemon juice
Organic red or black pepper
1–2 tsp. organic balsamic vinegar
Himalayan pink sea salt to taste

Put all vegetables in a bowl, pour the lemon juice and drizzle some balsamic vinegar and toss gently to mix. Add sea salt and pepper to taste, if desired.

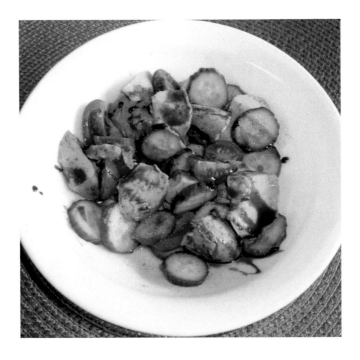

*Be sure to check the beginning of the book in the TIPS section for many helpful hints, alternatives, substitutes or suggestions that could save time and energy!*

# Asian Cabbage Salad

1/2 small head of organic cabbage, shredded
3/4 cup organic pea shoots, chopped
1 – 2 tbsp. organic sesame seeds, toasted if desired

*Serve with Asian Dressing, pg. 65*

Wash vegetables. Toss all together, add dressing and thoroughly mix. To toast sesame seeds; heat in a small saucepan on med-low for a few minutes until browning begins and remove quickly. Add seeds to salad and serve.

*Be sure to check the beginning of the book in the TIPS section for many helpful hints, alternatives, substitutes or suggestions that could save time and energy!*

# Cauliflower Salad

1 1/2 cup cauliflower, chopped small
1 cup organic kale, stem removed and chopped
2 stalk organic celery, chopped
1/2 cup sugar snap peas
1/2 cup grape tomato, cut in half
1/4 cup organic red onion, chopped
1 tsp. Himalayan pink sea salt and pepper to taste
2 tbsp. pumpkin seeds
2 tbsp. walnuts (whole or chopped)

*Serve with Balsamic Vinaigrette, pg. 66, or Hot-N-Spicy Balsamic, pg. 69*

Wash all vegetables. Chop cauliflower into small pieces. Remove stem from kale and chop. Cut celery and red onion into fine slices, chop snap peas and slice tomatoes in half. Add all ingredients in a bowl, add dressing salt pepper and toss all together to mix well. Let sit for 10-15 minutes before serving.

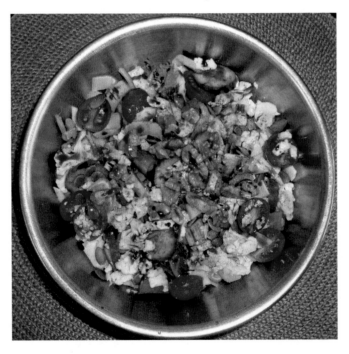

*Be sure to check the beginning of the book in the TIPS section for many helpful hints, alternatives, substitutes or suggestions that could save time and energy!*

# Baby Arugula Salad

1 bunch organic baby arugula
1/4 cup organic red onion, thinly sliced
1/2 cup organic cherry or grape tomatoes cut in half
1 stalk organic celery, thinly sliced
1/4 cup grated goat parmesan cheese, dairy-free cheese substitute or nutritional yeast
Himalayan pink sea salt and pepper to taste

*Serve with Mustard Dressing, pg. 73*

Wash vegetables. Wash arugula and spin to dry. Put all ingredients in a bowl. Mix dressing in a glass bottle with a pouring lid. Shake well before serving. Add enough dressing to blend and toss all together.

Optional: add sliced organic turkey or chicken strips.

*Be sure to check the beginning of the book in the TIPS section for many helpful hints, alternatives, substitutes or suggestions that could save time and energy!*

## Chickpea and Feta Salad

1 can organic chickpeas, rinsed and drained
1/3 cup goat's milk feta cheese, crumbled, dairy-free cheese substitute
or nutritional yeast
1/3 cup organic red onion, chopped
1/2 cup organic celery, chopped
1/2 cup organic english cucumber, sliced
Himalayan pink sea salt to taste
1 tbsp. fresh cilantro, chopped fine

*Serve with Apple Cider Vinaigrette, pg. 64*

Wash all vegetables. Add everything to a medium size bowl
and toss together to blend, top with crumbled feta or cheese
substitute. Add the dressing and stir, sprinkle chopped cilantro
and fresh ground sea salt and pepper to taste.

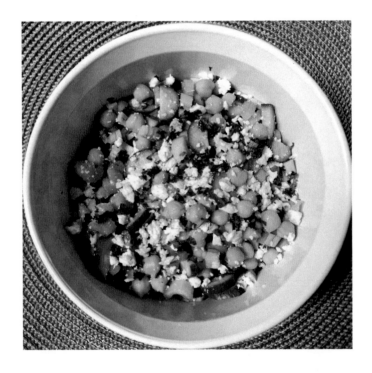

*Be sure to check the beginning of the book in the TIPS section for many helpful
hints, alternatives, substitutes or suggestions that could save time and energy!*

## Summer Berries Salad

1 avocado, medium size (not too ripe)
1/4 cup organic red onion, chopped fine
1/2 cup organic blackberries
1 cup organic raspberries or strawberries
1 cup organic blueberries
1/4 cup organic slivered almonds
1/4 cup organic raw pumpkin seeds
1/4 cup organic unsweetened shredded coconut
1/4 cup soft goat, vegan, dairy-free cheese substitute or nutritional yeast
2 tbsp. coconut vinegar
Drizzling of balsamic glaze

Wash all fruit and pat dry to remove excess water. Remove stone from avocado and cut in thin wedges or cubes then place in a medium size bowl. Add onion, berries, almonds, seeds and shredded coconut. Gently toss just enough to blend. Sprinkle the coconut vinegar all around the top then drizzle back and forth with the balsamic glaze.

Enjoy this delicious salad on a warm day with your favourite glass of Rose!

*Be sure to check the beginning of the book in the TIPS section for many helpful hints, alternatives, substitutes or suggestions that could save time and energy!*

# Iceberg and Avocado Salad

1 head organic iceberg lettuce washed and torn or cut
1/2 firm organic avocado, sliced
1 stalk organic celery, chopped
3/4 cup organic grape tomatoes
1/4 cup toasted pine nuts
1 tsp. Or 1 wedge of fresh lemon

*Serve with Balsamic Vinaigrette, pg. 66*

Wash lettuce and vegetables. Spin lettuce in salad spinner or roll in a towel and shake out excess water. Put torn lettuce in a large serving bowl; add celery, avocado slices and tomatoes. Squeeze the lemon over top of the avocado to prevent browning. Toast the pine nuts in a small frying pan on medium heat for about 10-15 minutes until lightly brown (no oil needed). Stir frequently to prevent burning.

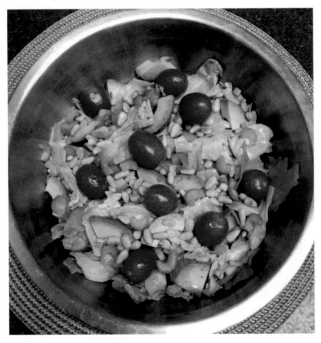

*Be sure to check the beginning of the book in the TIPS section for many helpful hints, alternatives, substitutes or suggestions that could save time and energy!*

## Beet Salad

1 med organic raw beet, peeled and sliced in thin strips
1 head organic iceberg lettuce, sliced in strips
1 cup organic english cucumber, sliced in strips

*Serve with Mustard Dressing, pg. 73*

Wash vegetables. Mix all together in a bowl and toss with dressing about 5 minutes before serving.

*Be sure to check the beginning of the book in the TIPS section for many helpful hints, alternatives, substitutes or suggestions that could save time and energy!*

## Quinoa and Chickpea Salad

1 cup quinoa, cooked
1 can organic chickpeas, drained
1–2 stalks organic celery, chopped
1/4 cup organic red onion, chopped small
1 half organic red, yellow or orange pepper, chopped small
1/2 cup organic soy or dairy-free mayonnaise substitute
1 tbsp. organic yellow mustard
1 tsp. Himalayan pink sea salt
1/2 tsp. cayenne pepper

Cook the quinoa as per the package instructions and let cool for about 30 minutes before mixing with other ingredients. In a large bowl add all other ingredients and slightly mix. Add cooled quinoa and mix thoroughly to blend all together.

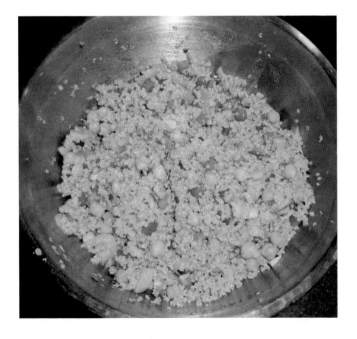

*Be sure to check the beginning of the book in the TIPS section for many helpful hints, alternatives, substitutes or suggestions that could save time and energy!*

## White Fish Wraps

White fish fillets
Brown rice tortillas or any gluten-free wrap of your choice
1 tbsp. lemon olive oil (or lemon juice and olive oil)
Organic mustard to taste
Organic soy mayonnaise or dairy-free mayonnaise substitute
Kale or spinach leaves

Steam the fish fillets in the same amount of lemon oil and water until cooked, approx 6 – 8 minutes. Wash, dry and tear the leaves. If using kale it may be desirable to remove the stem as it can be tough. Soften the brown rice tortilla shell and place on a piece of wax paper. Spread on desired amounts of mustard and soy mayonnaise; add the green leaves and fish. Roll up and fold in the bottom of the tortilla to keep contents intact.

Optional: substitute white fish for tilapia, basa, or haddock, if desired.

Place tortilla shells inside a foil sleeve and put in 250° oven for about 10 minutes to soften.
Wrap the wax paper around tightly with the top edges easy to peel away as you eat. This will make it less messy and keep your food inside.

*Be sure to check the beginning of the book in the TIPS section for many helpful hints, alternatives, substitutes or suggestions that could save time and energy!*

# Light Summer Salad

1 bunch organic red leaf lettuce
1/4 cup organic red onion, thinly sliced
2 stalks organic celery, chopped
1/2–3/4 cup organic cherry or grape tomatoes
2 tbsp. soft goat's milk cheese, crumbled, dairy-free cheese substitute or nutritional yeast
1/4 cup pine nuts, toasted (optional)
Himalayan pink sea salt to taste

*Serve with Balsamic Vinaigrette, pg. 66*

Add pine nuts to a small skillet on medium low heat. Stir or flip continually as they will toast very fast and can burn if not careful. Remove from heat once lightly browned. Wash vegetables and tear lettuce into pieces. Add the red onion slices, celery, tomatoes and toasted pine nuts. Crumble the goat or non-dairy cheese using a fork to scrape it onto the salad. Mix in dressing and a pinch of sea salt before serving.

*Be sure to check the beginning of the book in the TIPS section for many helpful hints, alternatives, substitutes or suggestions that could save time and energy!*

## Lentil Salad

1–19oz. can organic lentils, rinsed and drained
1 cup brown rice, cooked
2 cups organic red and yellow peppers, chopped fine
1/3 cup organic red onion, chopped fine
1/2 cup feta cheese, crumbled, dairy-free cheese substitute or nutritional yeast

Dressing:
3 tbsp. organic balsamic vinegar
2 cloves garlic, minced
1/2 tsp. cayenne pepper
3 tbsp. extra virgin organic olive oil

Combine cooked rice, lentils, chopped peppers, onions and feta cheese. Mix up the dressing and toss with other ingredients. It is best to refrigerate for 2-3 hours for flavours to blend. Stir together before serving.

*Be sure to check the beginning of the book in the TIPS section for many helpful hints, alternatives, substitutes or suggestions that could save time and energy!*

## Spinach Salad

1 bunch organic baby spinach
1/4 cup organic red onion, thinly sliced
1/2 cup organic grape tomatoes
1/2 cup organic cucumber, sliced
1/4 cup goat's milk feta cheese, dairy-free cheese substitute or
nutritional yeast

*Serve with Apple Cider Vinaigrette, pg. 64*

Wash spinach and spin to dry. Wash vegetables. Mix spinach,
onion, red pepper and celery together and top with crumbled
feta or substitute. Mix dressing ingredients in a glass bottle with
a pouring lid and shake to blend. Pour some dressing over salad
and mix before serving.
Optional: serve with a grilled salmon burger.

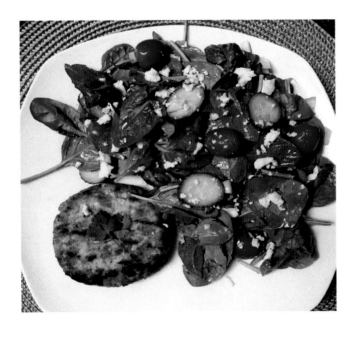

*Be sure to check the beginning of the book in the TIPS section for many helpful
hints, alternatives, substitutes or suggestions that could save time and energy!*

# Mix Your Favourite Greens Salad

Organic baby spinach
Organic arugula
Organic baby romaine
Organic red leaf
Organic green leaf
Organic endive
Organic swiss chard
Organic roasted red peppers, chopped
Organic avocado, sliced
1/3 cup slivered almonds, walnuts, or pine nuts, toasted

*\*Serve with Balsamic Vinaigrette, pg. 66*

Choose 3 or 4 different lettuces for variety, texture and appearance. Wash all lettuce and spin in a salad spinner or roll in a towel and refrigerate for crisping up to 1 hr ahead of time. Tear into bite size pieces, spin again or pat dry to ensure all excess water is removed. Put lettuce in large serving bowl; add chopped roasted peppers and avocado. Pine nuts can be toasted in a shallow baking sheet at 275° for 10–15 minutes until starting to brown, or turned in a small skillet on medium low heat. Toss bowl ingredients together gently, mix in some dressing, toss again and add the toasted pine nuts on top then serve in individual bowls.

*Be sure to check the beginning of the book in the TIPS section for many helpful hints, alternatives, substitutes or suggestions that could save time and energy!*

# Sweet Potato Salad

2 med organic sweet potato, skin on, cut in small cubes
1 stalk organic celery, chopped
1 small organic red onion, chopped fine
1 organic red pepper, chopped
1 1/2 cups organic broccoli, chopped small
1/2 can organic black beans, drained and rinsed
Himalayan pink sea salt and pepper to taste

*Creamy Dressing:*
2 tbsp. diary-free mayonnaise substitute
1 tsp. balsamic vinegar
1 tsp. lemon juice
Pinch of cayenne pepper (if desired)
Mix all together in a glass jar and pour on salad

Wash vegetables. Cook sweet potatoes until tender but not too soft then refrigerate to cool before cutting into cubes. Place all vegetables in a large bowl, mix in some creamy dressing and gently blend together until mixed through, adding more dressing if needed.

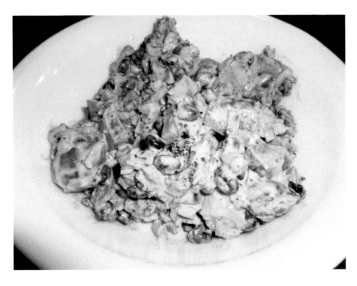

*Be sure to check the beginning of the book in the TIPS section for many helpful hints, alternatives, substitutes or suggestions that could save time and energy!*

# Super Greens Salad

3-4 leaves organic kale, stem removed and torn
4 leaves organic red leaf lettuce, torn
2 leaves organic swiss chard, torn
1/2 cup organic grape tomatoes
1/2 cup organic celery, sliced
1/4 cup organic red onion, sliced

Optional: add 1/2 cup raw organic pumpkin seeds

*Serve with Hot-N-Spicy Balsamic Dressing, pg. 69*

Wash vegetables. Wash all leaves well and spin to dry. Cut tomatoes in half. Chop onion in thin slivers. Add leaves to serving bowl and top with tomatoes, onions and seeds. Pour some dressing over salad and toss together before serving.

*Be sure to check the beginning of the book in the TIPS section for many helpful hints, alternatives, substitutes or suggestions that could save time and energy!*

# Walnut and Broccoli Salad

1/2 head organic iceberg lettuce, torn
3-4 large leaves organic kale, torn and stem removed
1 cup organic cherry or grape tomatoes
1/2 cup organic walnuts, chopped into large pieces
1/4 cup raw organic pumpkin seeds
1/4 cup organic goat cheddar cheese, dairy-free cheese substitute or nutritional yeast

*Serve with Balsamic Dijon Dressing, pg. 67*

Wash all vegetables. Toss all ingredients except the cheese in a large bowl. Add the dressing and blend until thoroughly mixed. Top with grated goat cheddar or substitute before serving.

*Be sure to check the beginning of the book in the TIPS section for many helpful hints, alternatives, substitutes or suggestions that could save time and energy!*

## Watermelon Salad

1 medium size watermelon, cut on chunks
1/2 cup goat feta cheese, cubed (omit if preferred)
1 cup organic cucumber, slivered
1 tbsp. fresh squeezed lemon juice
1 1/2 tbsp. extra virgin organic olive oil
3-4 fresh basil leaves, chopped fine
Dash of red or black pepper to taste

Mix watermelon and cucumber together in a large bowl, add the feta cheese and gently fold in. Squeeze the lemon juice all over and drizzle the olive oil on top. Garnish with the finely chopped basil and dash of ground red pepper. Let sit at room temperature for approx. 20 minutes before serving.

*Be sure to check the beginning of the book in the TIPS section for many helpful hints, alternatives, substitutes or suggestions that could save time and energy!*

# Vegetable Salad

1 organic English cucumber, cut in chunks or sliced
1 1/2 cups organic grape or cherry tomatoes
1/2 cup red onion, chopped fine
1 cup black olives
1 cup organic celery, sliced
1 small organic avocado, semi-firm, sliced in wedges
1/2 cup extra virgin organic olive oil
1/4 cup organic lemon juice, fresh squeezed
1 tsp. Himalayan pink sea salt
1/2 tsp. dried organic oregano or fresh basil, chopped
1 clove garlic, chopped

Mix all together and let sit for about 2 hours for all flavours to blend before serving.

*Be sure to check the beginning of the book in the TIPS section for many helpful hints, alternatives, substitutes or suggestions that could save time and energy!*

# DRESSINGS AND SAUCES

## Apple Cider Vinaigrette

1 tbsp. organic apple cider vinegar
1 tsp. organic fresh squeezed lemon juice
2 tsp. organic balsamic vinegar
3 tbsp. organic extra virgin olive oil

Mix in a glass bottle with a pouring lid. Shake well before serving.
Store in the fridge but be sure to let it reach room temperature
before serving.

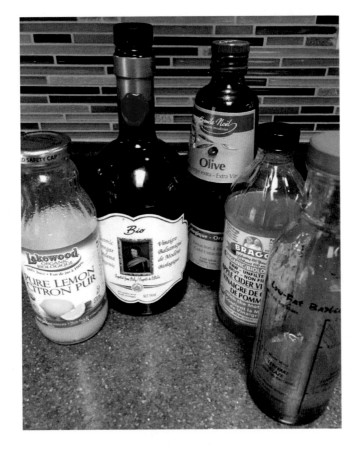

*Be sure to check the beginning of the book in the TIPS section for many helpful
hints, alternatives, substitutes or suggestions that could save time and energy!*

## Asian Dressing

1 tbsp. organic lemon, fresh squeezed
1 tbsp. organic sesame oil
1 tsp. organic tamari soy sauce
1 tsp. rice vinegar

Mix in a glass bottle with a pouring lid. Shake well before serving.
Store in the fridge.

*Be sure to check the beginning of the book in the TIPS section for many helpful hints, alternatives, substitutes or suggestions that could save time and energy!*

## Balsamic Vinaigrette

3 tbsp. organic balsamic vinegar
1 tsp. organic lemon juice
3 tbsp. organic extra virgin olive oil

Mix in a glass bottle with a pouring lid. Shake well before serving. Store in the fridge but be sure to let it reach room temperature before serving.

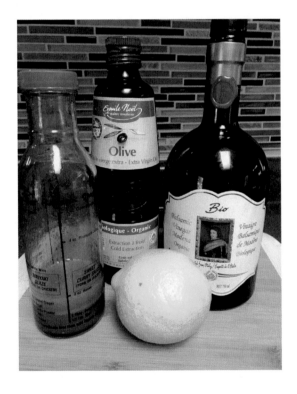

*Be sure to check the beginning of the book in the TIPS section for many helpful hints, alternatives, substitutes or suggestions that could save time and energy!*

# Balsamic Dijon Dressing

2 tbsp. organic balsamic vinegar
1 tsp. organic dijon mustard
1 tbsp. organic lemon juice
3 tbsp. organic extra virgin olive oil

Mix in a glass bottle with a pouring lid. Shake well before serving. Store in the fridge but be sure to let it reach room temperature before serving.

*Be sure to check the beginning of the book in the TIPS section for many helpful hints, alternatives, substitutes or suggestions that could save time and energy!*

# Lemon and Olive Oil Dressing

1 whole organic lemon, rolled and squeezed
2 tbsp. organic extra virgin olive oil
1 tsp. fresh parsley, chopped fine
1/2 tsp. lemon zest
Himalayan pink sea salt to taste

Wash the lemon with food wash. Roll on a cutting board or hard surface to soften and loosen the juices. Zest 1 tsp. of lemon peel and set aside. Cut the lemon and then squeeze through a strainer into a bowl. Mix all ingredients in a glass bottle with a pouring lid. Shake well before serving. Store in the fridge but be sure to let it reach room temperature before serving.

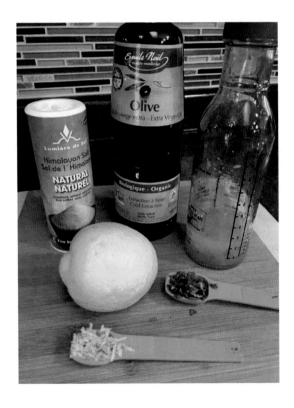

*Be sure to check the beginning of the book in the TIPS section for many helpful hints, alternatives, substitutes or suggestions that could save time and energy!*

# Hot-N-Spicy Balsamic Dressing

Add the following to the *Balsamic Vinaigrette, recipe on pg. 66* for a
hot-n-spicy variation
1/2 tsp. organic apple cider vinegar
1/2 tsp. cayenne pepper

Mix all ingredients in a glass bottle with a pouring lid. Shake to
blend well together. For sweeter taste add a bit of apple juice, for
hotter taste add more cayenne.

*Be sure to check the beginning of the book in the TIPS section for many helpful
hints, alternatives, substitutes or suggestions that could save time and energy!*

## Basic Red Sauce

4 cups fresh organic roma tomatoes, peeled and chopped OR
1 – 28 oz. can organic tomatoes, pureed in blender or food processor
8 oz. organic tomato juice
2 cloves organic garlic, minced
1 tbsp. organic extra virgin olive oil, grapeseed oil or avocado oil
1 tbsp. fresh oregano leaves, chopped fine (double if dried)
2 tbsp. fresh basil leaves, chopped fine (3 tbsp. if dried)
1/2 tsp. fresh ground sea salt
1/4 – 1/2 tsp. red or black pepper

Optional: add 1/2 cup Italian red wine (some good stuff: cook with the same wine you would drink!)

Puree tomatoes inside a large pot, add the olive oil, tomato juice, minced garlic oregano, basil and salt. Add wine if desired and cook over med heat for approx. 15 mins, then reduce to low heat for at least one hour.

Serve with any pasta or meat dish of your choice.

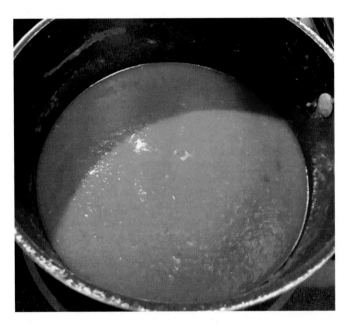

*Be sure to check the beginning of the book in the TIPS section for many helpful hints, alternatives, substitutes or suggestions that could save time and energy!*

# Red Wine Vinaigrette

1 tbsp. organic red wine vinegar
1 tsp. organic white wine vinegar
1/2 garlic bud squeezed or minced fine
2 tbsp. organic extra virgin olive oil

Mix in a glass bottle with a pouring lid. Shake well before serving. Store in the fridge but be sure to let it reach room temperature before serving.

*Be sure to check the beginning of the book in the TIPS section for many helpful hints, alternatives, substitutes or suggestions that could save time and energy!*

## Tahini Sauce

1/2 cup organic sesame paste
2 cloves garlic, mashed
1/3 cup organic lemon juice
1/4 cup organic extra virgin olive oil
1/2 tsp. Himalayan pink sea salt
1/4 cup water
1 tbsp. chopped cilantro

Mash garlic or chop very fine. Add all ingredients into a food processor and blend together until smooth and creamy.
Serve with falafels and sprinkle a bit of fresh cilantro on top.

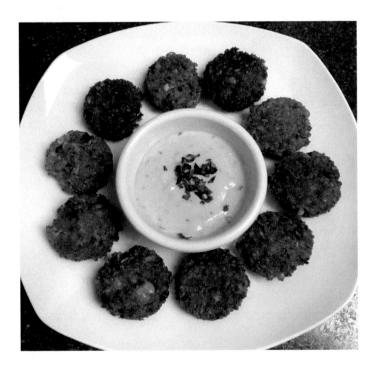

*Be sure to check the beginning of the book in the TIPS section for many helpful hints, alternatives, substitutes or suggestions that could save time and energy!*

# Mustard Dressing

2 tsp. organic balsamic vinegar
2 tsp. regular organic mustard
1 tsp. organic white wine vinegar
1 tsp. organic apple juice
2 tbsp. organic extra virgin olive oil
Himalayan pink sea salt to taste

Mix in a glass bottle with a pouring lid. Shake well before serving. Store in the fridge but be sure to let it reach room temperature before serving.

*Be sure to check the beginning of the book in the TIPS section for many helpful hints, alternatives, substitutes or suggestions that could save time and energy!*

# Fish Sauce

2 tbsp. organic prepared mustard
2 tbsp. soy mayonnaise or dairy-free mayonnaise substitute
1/2 organic lemon, squeezed
1/2 tsp. organic cayenne pepper
Dash of Himalayan pink sea salt

Mix all ingredients together and use as a baste as well as a dipping sauce for salmon, trout, white fish, tilapia or basa fillets.

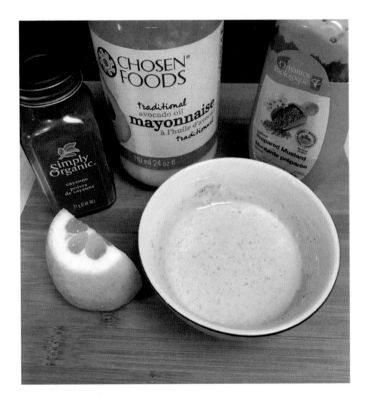

*Be sure to check the beginning of the book in the TIPS section for many helpful hints, alternatives, substitutes or suggestions that could save time and energy!*

# Coconut Curry Sauce

2 tbsp. organic extra virgin olive oil
1 tsp. crushed red chili pepper flakes
Zest of 1 organic lemon
1 1/2 tbsp. organic garlic, minced
1 –1 1/2 tbsp. curry powder
1 1/4 cup coconut milk
2 tbsp. gluten-free or coconut soy sauce
1/2 tsp. Himalayan pink sea salt
1/2 cup fresh basil leaves, chopped

Combine coconut milk, soy sauce, sea salt in small bowl. In skillet, add the oil and heat at medium-high for 30 seconds. Add pepper flakes, lemon zest, garlic and curry powder, stirring until fragrant, about 15 seconds. Add coconut milk mixture and bring to a boil. Cook until the sauce thickens slightly, about 2 minutes, and then add basil.
Serve with rice, green beans, tofu, or whatever you like.

Optional: substitute fresh cilantro for basil, if preferred.

*Be sure to check the beginning of the book in the TIPS section for many helpful hints, alternatives, substitutes or suggestions that could save time and energy!*

## Lemon Sauce

2 tbsp. extra virgin organic olive oil
1 whole organic lemon, squeezed
1 tbsp. zest of organic lemon
1/4 cup white wine
1 tsp. organic prepared mustard

Mix all ingredients in a bowl and whisk together to thoroughly blend.
Serve with any fish, rice, tofu or beef dish.

*Be sure to check the beginning of the book in the TIPS section for many helpful hints, alternatives, substitutes or suggestions that could save time and energy!*

# SOUPS

## Curried Squash Soup

1 butternut squash
1 organic bouillon cube; herb, onion or vegetable flavour
4 cups water
2 tbsp. coriander (cilantro) chopped fine
2 cloves garlic, minced
1/4 tsp. paprika
2 tsp. curry powder
1/2–3/4 soft mango (not ripe), cut in small cubes

Peel, seed and cut the squash in cubes. Dissolve the bouillon cube in 4 cups water, add the squash and bring to a boil. Reduce to simmer, add garlic, paprika and curry powder and cook for about 20 minutes uncovered. Use a hand mixer to blend in pot or transfer to a blender and blend until smooth and desired consistency is reached. Add the mango and simmer for another 10 minutes. Blend again until smooth or leave as is.

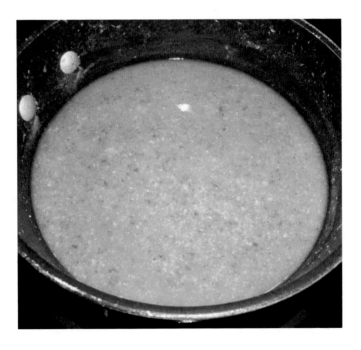

*Be sure to check the beginning of the book in the TIPS section for many helpful hints, alternatives, substitutes or suggestions that could save time and energy!*

# Pumpkin Soup

2 small-med sized cooking pumpkins
8 cups water
2 organic bouillon cubes; herb, onion or vegetable flavour
1 medium red onion, chopped
2 tbsp. grapeseed oil, avocado oil or organic extra virgin olive oil
1 tbsp. garlic, chopped fine
1/4 cup coriander (cilantro) chopped fine
2 tbsp. fresh squeezed lemon juice
1/2 tsp. cayenne pepper
1/2 tsp. paprika
1/2 tsp. Himalayan pink sea salt

Cut the pumpkins in half, remove seeds and place on a baking sheet lined with parchment paper; cook at 350° for approximately 35 minutes or until tender. In a large stock pot, heat the oil, add onion and cook for 5-10 minutes until tender. Add 4 cups water and bouillon cube, stirring to dissolve fully. Scoop the cooked pumpkin from the shell into the pot; add cayenne, paprika and garlic. Simmer covered for 30 minutes. Transfer to a blender in batches or use a hand mixer in the pot to blend until smooth. Add chopped cilantro, sea salt and lemon juice and heat for another 10 minutes.

Serve with garlic toast or crostini, if desired.

*Be sure to check the beginning of the book in the TIPS section for many helpful hints, alternatives, substitutes or suggestions that could save time and energy!*

## Sweet Potato and Squash Soup

| | |
|---|---|
| 1 large (2 1/2 cups) sweet potato | 1 tsp. cayenne pepper |
| 1 butternut squash | 1 tsp. Himalayan pink sea salt |
| 6 cups water | 1 med. onion, chopped small |

1 organic bouillon cube (vegetable, beef or chicken)
1 tbsp. grapeseed oil, avocado oil or organic extra virgin olive oil
1 tbsp. fresh chopped or dried cilantro or basil (if preferred)

Heat the oven to 350°. Cut the squash lengthwise and scoop out the seeds. Place the cut side down on a baking sheet lined with parchment paper and bake for approximately 35 – 40 minutes or until tender. In a large stock pot heat the oil and add the chopped onion. Cook onion until translucent, stirring often, add 6 cups of water and the bouillon cube, stirring until dissolved. Wash the sweet potato and cut in about 1-inch size pieces leaving skin on. Add to the pot and cook on med-high until potato is tender. Add the sea salt, herbs,and cayenne pepper. When squash is soft, remove from oven and scoop from skin in to the pot, reduce heat to simmer. Using a hand mixer, blend all together until smooth. If it is too thick some additional water can be added.
Top with finely grated parmesan or diary-free cheese substitute.

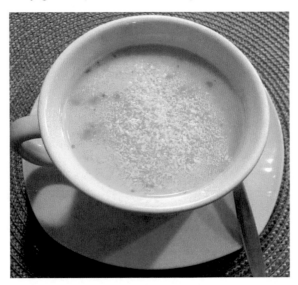

*Be sure to check the beginning of the book in the TIPS section for many helpful hints, alternatives, substitutes or suggestions that could save time and energy!*

# Harvest Soup

1 medium sweet potato
1 acorn squash
1 small cooking pumpkin
1 medium organic red onion, chopped small
8 cups water
1 organic bouillon cube (vegetable, beef or chicken)
1 tbsp. grapeseed oil, avocado oil or organic extra virgin olive oil
1 tsp. Himalayan pink sea salt
1 tsp. paprika pepper

Heat the oven to 350°. Cut the squash and pumpkin in half and scoop out the seeds. Place the cut side down on a baking sheet lined with parchment paper and bake for approximately 35 – 40 minutes or until a knife inserts easily. In a large stock pot heat the oil and add the chopped red onion. Cook onion until translucent, stirring often then add 8 cups of water and the bouillon cube, stirring until dissolved. Wash the sweet potato and cut in about 1-inch size pieces leaving skin on. Add to the pot and cook on med-high until potato is tender. Add the sea salt and paprika. When squash is soft, remove from oven and scoop from skin in to the pot, reduce heat to simmer. Using a hand mixer, blend all together until smooth. If it is too thick some additional water can be added.

Serve with a salad, crostini or crackers.

*Be sure to check the beginning of the book in the TIPS section for many helpful hints, alternatives, substitutes or suggestions that could save time and energy!*

# Cauliflower and Broccoli Soup

1 medium size cauliflower head, trimmed and chopped small
2 cups broccoli, chopped small
1 cup organic carrots, chopped small
2 cups curly kale, washed and chopped small
2 tbsp. grapeseed oil, avocado oil or organic extra virgin olive oil
1 medium size red onion, chopped fine
2 cloves garlic, minced
6 cups broth or water with organic veggie bouillon cube
1/2 – 1 tsp. Himalayan pink sea salt and pepper to taste
1 cup quinoa, rinsed

In a large stock pot, heat the oil, add onion and saute until soft and translucent. Add the stock or bouillon cube, dissolve in the water and stir to blend. Add all vegetables, minced garlic, salt and pepper. Heat at med-high for about 5 minutes with the lid on. Add the rinsed quinoa, and bring to a boil. Reduce to simmer and cook with the lid on for 15-20 minutes. Test vegetables for desired tenderness and continue to simmer.
Serve in individual bowls.

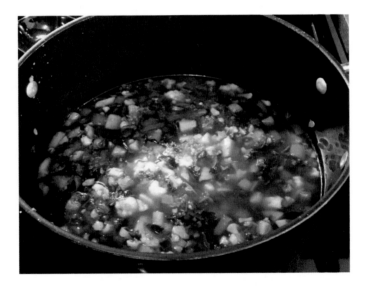

*Be sure to check the beginning of the book in the TIPS section for many helpful hints, alternatives, substitutes or suggestions that could save time and energy!*

# Bean Soup

1 can black bean
1 can chick peas
1 medium red onion
2 stalks celery, chopped
4 cups vegetable broth or bouillon cube
2 cloves garlic, minced
1 cup medium or mild Salsa
1 tsp. cayenne pepper
1 tbsp. grapeseed oil, avocado oil or organic extra virgin olive oil
1 tsp. Himalayan pink sea salt

Optional garnish: 1/2 cup shredded vegan cheese, goat marble or nutritional yeast.

Pour 1 tbsp. of oil in a stock pot and on medium heat, cook the onion until soft and transparent. Add the broth or bouillon cube dissolved in 4 cups of water and stir to blend. Add garlic, cayenne, sea salt, drained cans of beans and chick peas, stir together and heat for approx 15 minutes. Add the salsa and blend together. Add celery and simmer for about 5 minutes (longer if you don't want the celery crunchie). Serve right away.

Garnish with shredded cheese or nutritional yeast.

*Be sure to check the beginning of the book in the TIPS section for many helpful hints, alternatives, substitutes or suggestions that could save time and energy!*

# Roasted Red Pepper Soup

4 large sweet red peppers
1 tbsp. grapeseed oil, avocado oil or organic extra virgin olive oil
2 medium size red onion, chopped fine
2 cloves garlic, minced
5 cups broth (organic bouillon cube; chicken, beef or vegetable flavour)
2 tsp. paprika
1 tsp. organic honey
2 tbsp. fresh squeezed lemon juice
1/2 tsp. cayenne (optional)
Salt to taste – Himalayan pink sea salt

Place washed peppers on a baking sheet and roast in a 500° oven for about 20 minutes, turning occasionally until evenly charred. Remove from heat and cover over with an inverted bowl. Let stand for about 10 minutes. Working over a bowl, remove the skin reserving any juice but discarding stems and seeds. Cut peppers in approximate 1" strips. In a large stock pot, heat oil, add onions and cooks about 10 minutes, stirring often. Add peppers, their juice, garlic and 1 cup of water; cook uncovered for 10 minutes. Add broth, paprika, and honey; bring to a boil over med-hi heat. Reduce to simmer and cover for 20 minutes. Transfer soup to blender in batches or use a hand mixer in the pot to purée until smooth and desired consistency is reached. Add lemon juice, cayenne and sea salt to taste. Stir together and serve.

Serve with crostini or garlic pumpernickel cheese bread, if desired.

*Be sure to check the beginning of the book in the TIPS section for many helpful hints, alternatives, substitutes or suggestions that could save time and energy!*

# VEGETABLES AND GRAINS

## BBQ Veggies

1 organic sweet potato, slice and grill separately
1 cup organic cauliflower
1 cup organic broccoli
1 medium size organic red onion
1 cup organic brussel sprouts
1 cup organic asparagus
2 tbsp. organic balsamic vinegar
1 tbsp. organic extra virgin olive oil, grapeseed oil or avocado oil
1 clove organic garlic, minced or chopped fine

Clean all vegetables leaving skin on the sweet potato. Cut into large chunky pieces and toss together in a large bowl. In a small bowl, combine the vinegar, oil and minced garlic and stir until mixed. Pour over the vegetables, stir and let marinade for about 15 minutes. Using a grilling mat or BBQ basket, cook the vegetables at approx. 375°, turning often, until tender and browning.

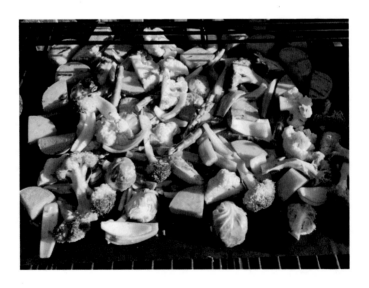

*Be sure to check the beginning of the book in the TIPS section for many helpful hints, alternatives, substitutes or suggestions that could save time and energy!*

# Basic Stir-fried Veggies

2 tsp. organic extra virgin olive oil, grapeseed oil or avocado oil
2 tsp. organic tamari soy sauce
2 tsp. organic lemon juice
1 med organic red onion, chopped
1 cup organic asparagus, cut into pieces
1 cup organic broccoli, cut into pieces
2 stalks organic celery, chopped
2-3 leaves organic kale, chopped with or without stem
3/4 cup organic cherry or grape tomatoes

Wash all vegetables. Heat olive oil in large stir fry pan. Add onion, broccoli and celery and cook for approx 5–7 minutes. Add asparagus and kale and continue to cook until all vegetables are tender but not soft, stirring frequently. Add tomatoes and tamari soy sauce and gently toss together. Remove from heat, pour lemon juice all over and serve. Try this with grilled salmon and your favorite rice or quinoa.

*Be sure to check the beginning of the book in the TIPS section for many helpful hints, alternatives, substitutes or suggestions that could save time and energy!*

## Best Red Rice

1 cup organic brown rice or organic brown basmati
2 cups organic tomato juice
3/4 cup organic celery, chopped
Pinch of sea salt to taste
Stove top or in the rice cooker

Wash vegetables. Substitute the suggested water amount for organic tomato juice, add the celery and sea salt. Cook as per the instructions for the method of cooking selected and add another 10 minutes.

*Be sure to check the beginning of the book in the TIPS section for many helpful hints, alternatives, substitutes or suggestions that could save time and energy!*

## Brown Basmati Rice

1 cup organic brown basmati rice
1/2 tsp. paprika
1/2 tsp. parsley flakes
1 1/2 tsp. fresh lemon juice
1 tsp. roasted garlic, finely chopped
2 cups water

Add all ingredients to a medium size pot. Bring to a boil, reduce heat to simmer, cover and cook for 50 minutes. Remove from heat and let stand for 5-7 minutes before serving.

*Be sure to check the beginning of the book in the TIPS section for many helpful hints, alternatives, substitutes or suggestions that could save time and energy!*

## Cauliflower Rice

1 medium cauliflower, washed and chopped fine
1/2 onion (red or white) diced small
1 – 2 tbsp. grapeseed or avocado oil

Wash and trim the center and leaves from the cauliflower. Dry off excess water. Cut in half, then into smaller florets. Use a food processor or chopper and chop (in batches) until small granules. Dice onion very small. Heat 1 tbsp. oil in sauce pan on medium heat. Add onion and saute a couple minutes, until translucent. Add cauliflower (more oil if needed), cover and cook for approx. 5 – 8 minutes until tender but not soft.

Serve immediately. Can be stored in the fridge for up to a week.

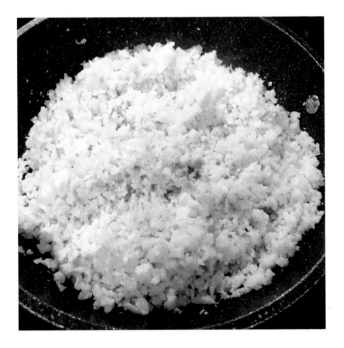

*Be sure to check the beginning of the book in the TIPS section for many helpful hints, alternatives, substitutes or suggestions that could save time and energy!*

# Green Vegetable Stir-fry

1 1/2 cups organic green beans, cut in half
2 stalks organic celery, cut in large pieces
8-10 leaves organic beet tops or swiss chard, cut
1 half organic yellow pepper, cut in large pieces
1 tbsp. organic roasted garlic, minced
1/3 cup pine nuts
2 tsp. organic extra virgin olive oil, grapeseed oil or avocado oil
Fresh ground sea salt

Wash vegetables. Heat pan, add oil; add beans, celery and pepper and sauté for about 5 minutes. Add beet tops and garlic, continuing to cook until tender. When almost done, make a well in the middle and add the pine nuts, turning often to brown but do not burn. Add some fresh ground sea salt before serving.

*Be sure to check the beginning of the book in the TIPS section for many helpful hints, alternatives, substitutes or suggestions that could save time and energy!*

## Lemon Brown Basmati Rice

1 cup organic brown basmati rice
2 cups water
2 tbsp. fresh organic lemon juice
1 tsp. organic parsley flakes

Put all ingredients in a med size pot and bring to a boil. Cover and simmer for 50 minutes, remove from heat and let stand for 5–7 minutes. Serve with steamed broccoli, asparagus, kale or spinach.

*Be sure to check the beginning of the book in the TIPS section for many helpful hints, alternatives, substitutes or suggestions that could save time and energy!*

# Peppery Hot Stir-fry Veggies

1 whole raw organic beet, peeled and thinly sliced into sticks
1 cup organic swiss chard, chopped
1 cup organic spinach, chopped
1/2 cup organic celery, chopped
1/2 cup organic asparagus, chopped
1 cup partially cooked organic sweet potato, skin on, chopped
1 tsp. organic extra virgin olive oil, grapeseed oil or avocado oil
1 tsp. organic hot pepper oil or chili pepper oil
1 tsp. organic garlic, minced

Thoroughly wash all vegetables before chopping. Pour 1 tbsp. of water into frying pan, add all vegetables and steam before flying. When water is evaporated; add olive oil, hot pepper oil and stir fry veggies on medium until browning. Serve with organic brown rice and your favorite fish.

Optional: fresh chopped chili peppers can be substituted for the pepper oil, but add more olive oil if substituting.

*Be sure to check the beginning of the book in the TIPS section for many helpful hints, alternatives, substitutes or suggestions that could save time and energy!*

## Quinoa with Nuts and Cheese

1 cup organic quinoa
2 tbsp. soft plain goat cheese, dairy-free cheese substitute or nutritional yeast
1/2 cup organic celery, chopped
1/2 cup organic walnuts, finely chopped (optional)
1/2 tsp. Himalayan pink sea salt
Black or red pepper to taste

Rinse quinoa well for 3–5 minutes and drain. Wash vegetables. Add to 2 cups of water in a medium sized pot. Bring to a boil and reduce heat to simmer, cover and let cook for 11–15 minutes. Quinoa is done when it is transparent and all water is absorbed. Add the goat cheese or non-dairy cheese, celery and walnuts if desired. Quinoa has a nutty flavour on its own which can be enhanced by adding walnuts.

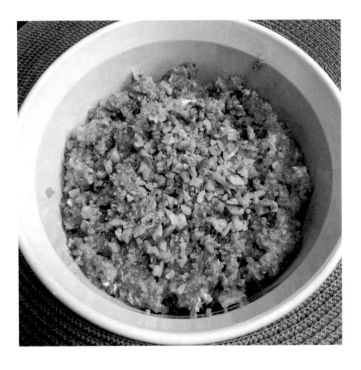

*Be sure to check the beginning of the book in the TIPS section for many helpful hints, alternatives, substitutes or suggestions that could save time and energy!*

# Quick Spicy Rice

1 cup organic brown rice
1/2 cup organic hot salsa

Cook the rice as per instructions for stove top or rice cooker. Mix in salsa and heat through then serve.

Optional: substitute brown rice for brown basmati or your favorite rice, if preferred.
Optional: substitute the hot salsa for medium or mild, if preferred.

*Be sure to check the beginning of the book in the TIPS section for many helpful hints, alternatives, substitutes or suggestions that could save time and energy!*

## Stir-fry with Nuts

2 stalks organic celery, chopped
1 med organic green pepper, cut in strips
1 med organic red onion, cut in thin strips
3/4 cup organic grape tomatoes
1/2 cup pine nuts
1-2 tsp. organic soy sauce (or soy alternative)
2 tsp. organic extra virgin olive oil, grapeseed oil or avocado oil

Wash all vegetables. Heat pan and add olive oil; add veggies except tomatoes and sauté over med heat until starting to brown and soften. Add tomatoes and soy sauce and cook approx 5 minutes. Make a well in the middle of pan and add the pine nuts, stirring often until they start to brown. Remove and serve.

*Be sure to check the beginning of the book in the TIPS section for many helpful hints, alternatives, substitutes or suggestions that could save time and energy!*

## Quinoa with Peas

1 cup organic quinoa
2 cups water
3/4 cup organic celery, chopped
1 cup organic peas, fresh or frozen
1 tbsp. organic roasted garlic, chopped

Wash vegetables. Rinse quinoa for 3–5 minutes, add to boiling water and bring to a boil. Reduce to simmer, cover and cook for 8–10 minutes. Add peas and cook for another 5 minutes or until all moisture is absorbed.

*Be sure to check the beginning of the book in the TIPS section for many helpful hints, alternatives, substitutes or suggestions that could save time and energy!*

# Roasted Sweet Potato and Walnuts

4 cups sweet potato, washed and cut in chunks
1 small vidalia or sweet onion, cut in chunks
2 cloves garlic, chopped fine
3 tbsp. organic extra virgin olive oil, grapeseed oil or avocado oil
1 tsp. dried or fresh thyme
1/2 cup walnuts, halved
1 tbsp. balsamic vinegar or balsamic glaze
Fresh ground Himalayan pink sea salt and pepper to taste

In a large bowl combine the sweet potato, onion, garlic, oil and thyme. Toss together to coat then place in a shallow baking dish. Bake at 425° turning frequently for 40–45 minutes or until soft. At the last 10 minutes, add the nuts and drizzle with balsamic vinegar, sea salt and pepper to taste.

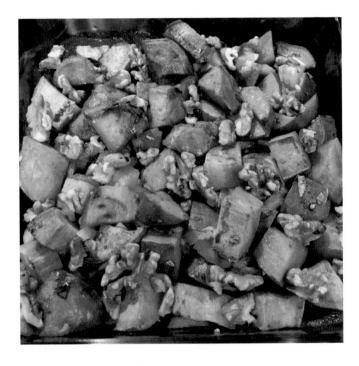

*Be sure to check the beginning of the book in the TIPS section for many helpful hints, alternatives, substitutes or suggestions that could save time and energy!*

## Roasted Red Peppers

6-8 organic red peppers (at a time)

Heat the oven to 400°. Wash and pat dry the peppers. Place on a cookie sheet. Cook for 20 minutes, turn and roast another 20 minutes. Remove from oven and place in a large zip-lock bag to sweat for 20 minutes. Peel skin easily, remove seeds and stem. Cut and use for salads, antipasto, sandwiches, omelets, pasta, etc. or simply enjoy as they are with some drizzled olive oil.

*Be sure to check the beginning of the book in the TIPS section for many helpful hints, alternatives, substitutes or suggestions that could save time and energy!*

## Quinoa with Spinach

1 cup organic quinoa
3/4 cup organic spinach, chopped
1/4 cup organic celery, chopped
1/4 cup organic red onion, chopped
2 cups water

Wash vegetables. Rinse quinoa for approx 3–5 minutes. Put all ingredients into a med size pot and bring to a boil. Reduce to simmer, cover and cook for 10–12 minutes or until all water is evaporated.

*Be sure to check the beginning of the book in the TIPS section for many helpful hints, alternatives, substitutes or suggestions that could save time and energy!*

# Sweet and Hot Brown Rice

1 cup organic brown rice, rinsed
1/3 cup organic broccoli stems, chopped and peeled
1/3 cup organic celery, chopped fine
1/4 cup hot chile peppers, chopped fine
1 small organic sweet potato
1 tbsp. organic pure maple syrup
1/8 tsp. Himalayan pink sea salt

Wash all vegetables and scrub sweet potato with skin on. Cook until tender and set aside to cool before cutting. Put rice and 2 cups water in a med pot and bring to a boil. Cover, reduce to simmer and cook for 40 minutes. Cut the sweet potato into small pieces. Remove from heat and let stand for 5 minutes. Add broccoli stems, celery, sweet and hot peppers, return to simmer covered for 5–10 minutes then remove from heat, add maple syrup and sea salt and mix together. Serve with fish, pork or beef.

*Be sure to check the beginning of the book in the TIPS section for many helpful hints, alternatives, substitutes or suggestions that could save time and energy!*

# Sautéed Broccoli and Cabbage

1 1/2 cups organic broccoli with stems, chopped thin
1 1/2 cups yellow cabbage, shredded
1/2 cup red onion, chopped fine
3 - 4 beet top leaves with stems, chopped
2 tbsp. organic extra virgin olive oil, grapeseed oil or avocado oil
2 tbsp. slivered almonds, chopped
Fresh ground Himalayan pink sea salt and pepper to taste

Wash all vegetables and trim broccoli and beet tops. Shred cabbage with a grater. Chop the onion in small slivers. Chop broccoli in thin slices and chop stem of beet tops into small pieces. Heat the oil in the pan on medium, add the onion, broccoli, cabbage and beet stems. Saute until tender, stirring often, add the beet tops and continue to cook. Grind some fresh sea salt and pepper on top, reduce heat if it gets too hot and add the chopped almonds just before serving. Toss altogether to mix well and serve.

Optional: substitute beet tops with spinach, if preferred.

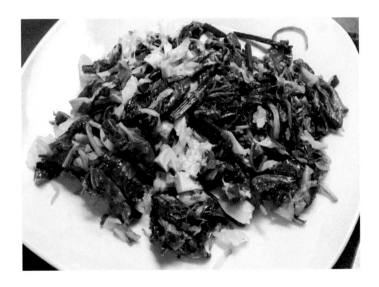

*Be sure to check the beginning of the book in the TIPS section for many helpful hints, alternatives, substitutes or suggestions that could save time and energy!*

## Tomato Quinoa

1/2 medium organic onion, chopped fine
1 tbsp. organic extra virgin olive oil, grapeseed oil or avocado oil
1 1/2 tbsp. fresh organic cilantro, chopped
1 cup organic quinoa, rinsed
1 cup water
1 cup organic roma tomatoes, pureed

Heat oil in medium sized pot, add onions and cook for about 5 minutes. Add chopped cilantro, water, tomato and quinoa. Bring to a boil, reduce to simmer, cover and cook 12–15 minutes or until all water is absorbed.

*Be sure to check the beginning of the book in the TIPS section for many helpful hints, alternatives, substitutes or suggestions that could save time and energy!*

## Zucchini Meat Balls

2 organic zucchini, chopped
1/2 cup red onion, chopped
1/4 organic spinach, chopped fine
2 tbsp. egg whites
1 large clove garlic, mashed
1/3 cup organic goat feta cheese, dairy-free cheese substitute or nutritional yeast
1-2 tsp. dried chili peppers
2 tbsp. organic sun-dried tomato, softened and chopped
1/2 cup organic chick peas, cooked and mashed
2 tbsp. ground almonds
4-6 leaves fresh basil, chopped
2/3 cup amaranth flour
2 tbsp. organic extra virgin olive oil, grapeseed oil or avocado oil

Boil the chopped zucchini and onion to soften then drain well. Mash the zucchini and onion together in a large bowl. Add the flour, mashed chick peas, spinach, almonds and egg whites and blend together. Add all remaining ingredients other than oil and blend all together well. Form into round balls and then cook in oil over medium heat, turning gently to cook all sides until crispy.

*Be sure to check the beginning of the book in the TIPS section for many helpful hints, alternatives, substitutes or suggestions that could save time and energy!*

# MAIN COURSE

# BBQ Fish and Grilled Vegetables

2 White fish fillets (fresh or frozen) defrosted
1/2 organic cauliflower, cut in florets
1/2 organic broccoli, cut in florets
1 cup organic asparagus, ends snapped off
3 stalks organic celery, cut in large pieces
1 organic red pepper, cut in large slices
Extra virgin olive oil, grapeseed oil or avocado oil
Organic balsamic vinegar
Fresh lemon
Fine chopped fresh basil (optional)

Wash and cut all vegetables into large pieces appropriate for grilling. Toss in a large bowl with the oil and balsamic vinegar. Put vegetables in a grilling bowl or on a grilling pad and cook for approx 10–15 minutes on medium heat turning often. Lightly brush fish with olive oil on each side and use a fish grilling pan, gilling pad or place fish on foil. Grill fish for 5–7 minutes each side for thick fillets (less is thin). Squeeze half of a fresh lemon on the fillets when they are first removed from the grill and season with fresh ground sea salt and pepper if desired.

Optional: add fresh chopped basil or cilantro before grilling.
Optional: White fish could be tilapia, basa, cod or haddock.

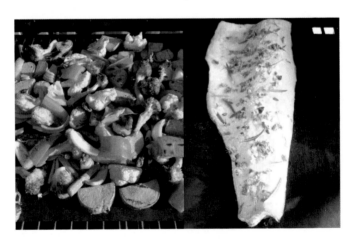

*Be sure to check the beginning of the book in the TIPS section for many helpful hints, alternatives, substitutes or suggestions that could save time and energy!*

# BBQ Wild Salmon and Vegetables

2 wild salmon fillets
1 med organic eggplant, sliced thick
1 organic pepper (yellow/red/purple/orange), sliced thick
1 cup organic beans (yellow/green/purple), ends trimmed
1 cup asparagus, ends snapped off
1/2 cup goat's milk feta cheese, dairy-free cheese substitute or
nutritional yeast

*Balsamic Vinaigrette, recipe on pg. 66*

Heat BBQ and set at medium temperature. Wash vegetables.
An easy way to cut off the correct amount of asparagus stem is
to hold the very bottom in two fingers and bend until the stem
snaps. It will break off exactly the amount needed. Lightly brush
the salmon fillets with organic extra virgin olive oil. Toss the cut
vegetables in 2 tbsp. of *balsamic vinaigrette before cooking in
a grilling bowl on the top shelf of the BBQ. Cook approx 5–10
minutes turning often. Place the Wild Salmon skin side up on the
grill and cook for 3 minutes. Turn over and cook skin side down for
7 minutes. Do not over cook. Remove vegetables from grill and
toss in crumbled goat feta before serving. Serve with baked sweet
potato if desired.

*Be sure to check the beginning of the book in the TIPS section for many helpful
hints, alternatives, substitutes or suggestions that could save time and energy!*

# BBQ Turkey Breast

1 1/4 cup each serving boneless skinless organic turkey breasts
(substitute chicken if desired)
1 tbsp. *balsamic Vinaigrette, recipe on pg. 66
1 organic zucchini, sliced thick
1 organic eggplant, sliced thick

Wash and cut the zucchini and eggplant into slices that are
suitable for grilling. Toss in a stainless bowl with some balsamic
vinaigrette. Brush the turkey breasts with balsamic vinaigrette and
let sit for about 10 minutes before grilling. Heat the BBQ to about
375°. Using a grilling mat, cook the veggies for about 5 minutes,
turning often. Add the turkey breasts and cook for approx. 10
minutes each side (dependent on the size of each breast), adjust
for thickness.

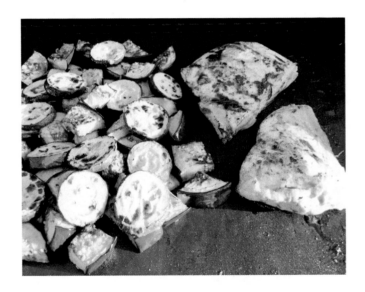

*Be sure to check the beginning of the book in the TIPS section for many helpful
hints, alternatives, substitutes or suggestions that could save time and energy!*

## Baked Cod Fish

2 organic cod fish fillets, frozen is best
1 fresh organic lemon
Himalayan pink sea salt
Black or cayenne pepper to taste

Wash organic lemon before cutting. Place frozen fillets in a shallow non-stick baking dish. Slice half the lemon in thin slices and place on top of the fillets and/or squeeze fresh juice on fish. Add a light dusting of sea salt and pepper (if desired). Cover with lid or foil and bake at 375° for 8–10 minutes. If fish is thawed it will take less time.

Optional: Add some fresh chopped organic herbs like coriander, thyme, parsley or basil for additional seasoning.

Optional: fish can be tilapia, basa or haddock.

*Be sure to check the beginning of the book in the TIPS section for many helpful hints, alternatives, substitutes or suggestions that could save time and energy!*

# Baked Rainbow Trout

1-2 fillets – skinned and washed
2–3 tbsp. organic onion – finely chopped
Organic extra virgin olive oil, grapeseed oil or avocado oil

Sauce:
1 tbsp. organic brown mustard
1 tsp. organic stone ground mustard
1 tsp. organic dijon mustard
1 1/2 tsp. whole grain and seed mustard
1 1/2 tbsp. dairy-free mayonnaise or mayonnaise substitute
1 tsp. Braggs all purpose liquid soy seasoning
1/8 tsp. cayenne pepper
1/2 tsp. organic lemon juice

Mix all together and whisk until well blended and smooth.
Rinse fillets and pat dry with paper towel to remove excess water. Heat
broiler to high temperature or 500°. Spray a light coating of oil in a
baking dish or cookie sheet. Place fillets in the dish. Spoon the sauce
over the fish and spread enough to totally cover. Reserve some sauce for
serving. Sprinkle the finely chopped onion over each fillet. Broil on top
shelf for approx 6- 8 minutes, until fish is bubbling and starts to separate.
(Time may need to be adjusted for varying size of fillets). Let sit for 5
minutes before serving. Drizzle some of the reserved sauce if desired.

Optional: substitute for white fish, orange roughy or tilapia.

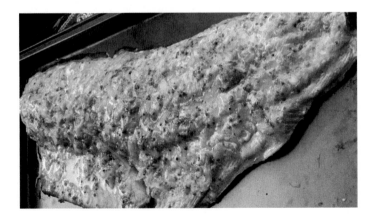

*Be sure to check the beginning of the book in the TIPS section for many helpful
hints, alternatives, substitutes or suggestions that could save time and energy!*

## Battered Fried Fish

2 large organic white fish fillets
1/2 cup rice or cashew milk
3/4 cup organic brown rice flour
1 tbsp. organic extra virgin olive oil, grapeseed oil or avocado oil
1 tbsp. organic fresh lemon juice

Fish Dip: mix 1 tbsp. organic mustard with 1 tbsp. organic soy-based mayonnaise substitute. To spice it up add 1/8 tsp. of cayenne pepper.

Wash fish and cut into strips like fingers. Dip into milk then coat with brown rice flour. Fry in heated pan with olive oil on med heat for 3–4 minutes and flip over. Squeeze fresh organic lemon juice over fish before serving.

Optional: substitute brown rice flour for organic almond flour to give a bit of a nutty flavour.
Optional: white fish could be tilapia, basa, cod or haddock.

*Be sure to check the beginning of the book in the TIPS section for many helpful hints, alternatives, substitutes or suggestions that could save time and energy!*

# Buffalo Stew

1 lb organic buffalo stewing meat
3 cups organic roma tomatoes, skin removed and chopped
1 tbsp. fresh basil, chopped fine
1 tsp. organic all-purpose seasoning
1 cup quinoa, rinsed
1 cup water
1 tsp. organic garlic, chopped
3 stalks organic celery, chopped
1 red sheppard pepper, chopped

Wash vegetables. Put tomatoes in large pot on medium heat, add basil and seasoning. Add a light spray of oil to a medium sized non-stick frying pan and heat to med- hi. Add the stewing meat and turn often to just brown on all sides. Add the meat to the tomatoes, cover and cook on med-lo for about 10 minutes then reduce to simmer for 50 minutes. Rinse the quinoa for 3 minutes and add to the pot as well as the chopped celery, peppers and garlic. Add the water, bring to a boil and reduce to simmer for 40 minutes. Check periodically to see if more liquid is needed and add either water or organic tomato juice as necessary. If tomatoes were frozen less water may be needed. Individual servings can be seasoned with sea salt and pepper if desired.

Optional: turn up the heat by adding 1 tsp. of cayenne pepper.
Optional: substitute beef or chicken for buffalo, if preferred.

*Be sure to check the beginning of the book in the TIPS section for many helpful hints, alternatives, substitutes or suggestions that could save time and energy!*

# Chickpea Stew

1–19oz. can organic chick peas
1 organic red pepper, chopped
1 organic zucchini, chopped
1 med organic red onion, chopped small
2 stalks organic celery, chopped
6–8 leaves organic spinach, chopped
1 med organic sweet potato, scrubbed, skin on chopped small
1–28oz. can organic tomatoes
1/8 tsp. cayenne pepper

Drain and rinse chick peas. Wash vegetables. Add canned tomatoes to a large pot and puree with hand blender to smooth out most of the lumps. Add all ingredients other than the cayenne to the pot and cook on med heat for 20 minutes. Reduce to simmer adding the cayenne and continue to cook for 30 minutes.

*Be sure to check the beginning of the book in the TIPS section for many helpful hints, alternatives, substitutes or suggestions that could save time and energy!*

## Easy Cheesy Pasta

Pasta - brown rice, quinoa, black bean or your preference
*Basic Red Sauce, recipe on pg. 70*
1/2 cup grated goat or sheep parmesan or dairy-free cheese substitute
1/4 cup soft goat's milk cheese or dairy-free cheese substitute, or nutritional yeast
Himalayan pink sea salt and red or black pepper to taste
Organic extra virgin olive oil

Prepare pasta, as per the package instructions.
When sauce is cooked and ready to serve, add desired cheese or nutritional yeast and stir until melted and mixed in. Serve on individual plates and drizzle a touch of olive oil over top.

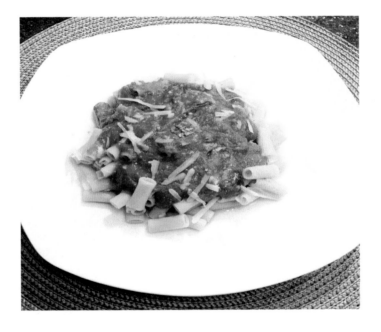

*Be sure to check the beginning of the book in the TIPS section for many helpful hints, alternatives, substitutes or suggestions that could save time and energy!*

# Ground Turkey with Salsa

1 lb. organic ground turkey
3 shakes cayenne pepper to taste
1/2 cup organic hot salsa

Cook ground turkey in a non-stick pan adding a few drops of extra virgin olive oil, grapeseed oil or avocado oil if needed to prevent sticking and break up in small bite size pieces. Add cayenne pepper and salsa, mix well.
Serve with cooked organic spinach and organic quinoa as a meal or mix all together and stuff in a wrap.

Optional: increase or decrease the cayenne to suit your own taste.
Optional: substitute hot salsa for medium or mild, if preferred.

*Be sure to check the beginning of the book in the TIPS section for many helpful hints, alternatives, substitutes or suggestions that could save time and energy!*

# Curried Vegetable Stew

3 tbsp. avocado oil
1 tsp. ground cayenne pepper
2 tbsp. yellow curry powder
2 tsp. Himalayan sea salt
1 med. organic onion, chopped
2 cans organic garbanzo beans

¼ cup fresh cilantro leaves
1 med. butternut squash
3 med. organic sweet potatoes
4 cups organic vegetable broth
1/2 head cauliflower, chopped

Wash the squash and sweet potato. Cut the squash in half lengthwise and remove the seeds. With skin on, cut the sweet potato lengthwise in half and half again. Place the squash and sweet potato on a cookie sheet lined with parchment paper. Bake at 350° for approx. 30 min or until just tender. Remove for the oven and cool 15 minutes then remove the skin from the squash and cut into bite size pieces. Cut the sweet potato into bite size pieces as well.

Heat the avocado oil and cayenne pepper in a large pot over medium heat add the onion and sauté until tender. Season with curry powder and salt and stir together cooking for a few minutes. Pour in the broth, and mix in the cauliflower. Bring to a boil, reduce heat to low, add the cut squash, sweet potatoes and stir. Partially mash the garbanzo beans with a fork, and add to the pot. Finely chop about 1 tbsp. of fresh cilantro and add to the pot and simmer 20–30 minutes. Serve in individual bowls and garnish with cilantro.

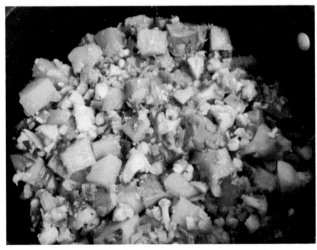

*Be sure to check the beginning of the book in the TIPS section for many helpful hints, alternatives, substitutes or suggestions that could save time and energy!*

## Lamb Steak – Broiled

2 lamb steaks (or thick chops)
1 tbsp. organic dijon mustard
1 tbsp. organic stone ground (or regular) mustard
2 cloves organic garlic
2 tsp. fresh cilantro chopped fine (optional)
2 tsp. organic apple cider vinegar
2 tsp. fresh basil, chopped fine
1 tsp. organic lemon juice
1 tsp. organic Worcestershire sauce
1/4 tsp. organic cayenne pepper

Mix all sauce ingredients together in a bowl. Place the lamb steaks in a glass baking dish. Preheat the oven to broil at high temperature. Spoon some sauce over the steaks, enough to cover. Broil for 5–7 minutes, turn over and add more sauce to the other side. Return to broil for 5–7 more minutes. Remove for the oven, cover with foil and let rest for 5 minutes before serving.

Serve with rice or quinoa and your choice of vegetables. Add any remaining sauce to meat or vegetables, if desired.

*Be sure to check the beginning of the book in the TIPS section for many helpful hints, alternatives, substitutes or suggestions that could save time and energy!*

# Pan Seared White Fish

Fresh or frozen white fish fillets, defrosted
1–2 tsp. organic extra virgin olive oil, grapeseed oil or avocado oil
1/4 cup organic red onion, chopped fine
Fresh sprig of herbs – thyme or rosemary
1 tbsp. fresh squeezed organic lemon juice

Rinse fish in cool water and pat dry. Finely chop the onion and the herbs. Heat oil in pan, place fillets in pan skin side up and squeeze some lemon juice over top. Cook over med heat for approx 2 minutes and carefully flip over. Spread the onion and herb on top of the fish, squeeze more lemon juice and cover with a lid for 2 minutes, then cook uncovered 3-5 minutes or until starting to separate. Remove from pan and serve with *lemon brown basmati rice (see recipe on page 92)* and steamed vegetables.

Optional: substitute for tilapia or trout.

*Be sure to check the beginning of the book in the TIPS section for many helpful hints, alternatives, substitutes or suggestions that could save time and energy!*

## Rice Vermicelli – Fried

Rice vermicelli
1 tbsp. organic extra virgin olive oil, grapeseed oil or avocado oil
2 tsp. organic soy sauce
1 cup cooked turkey, cut in strips

Add 2 servings vermicelli to boiling water and cook for 1 minute; quick rinse and drain well. Toss in 2 teaspoons olive oil and soy sauce and drop into heated frying pan with remaining olive oil. Fry for approximately 3 minutes turning often. Add the turkey strips and heat until warm. Serve with stir fried veggies and Asian cabbage salad.

Optional: substitute turkey for beef, if preferred.

*Be sure to check the beginning of the book in the TIPS section for many helpful hints, alternatives, substitutes or suggestions that could save time and energy!*

# Poached Fish in White Wine and Garlic

1 fish fillet (tilapia, basa, trout, haddock)
1–2 tsp. organic extra virgin olive oil, grapeseed oil or avocado oil
2 cloves garlic, chopped
1 tbsp. cilantro, chopped fine
1/2 organic lemon
2 tbsp. white wine

Heat the oil in a saucepan on medium; add garlic, cilantro and squeezed lemon juice and heat for about 5 minutes. Add the white wine and cover with a lid for 2 minutes. Add the fish fillet and cover, poaching the fish for about 5 minutes. Flip gently, reduce heat to low, cover and cook for a few more minutes until it starts to flake or separate. Don't overcook. Spoon some sauce over fish when serving. Garnish with some fresh cilantro. Cooking time may vary depending on the thickness of the fillet.

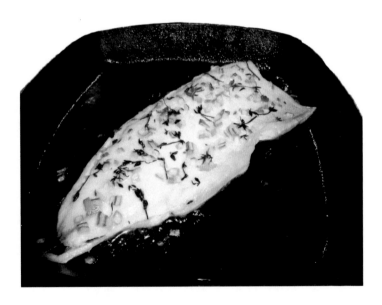

*Be sure to check the beginning of the book in the TIPS section for many helpful hints, alternatives, substitutes or suggestions that could save time and energy!*

# Gluten-free Pasta with Basic Red Sauce

Organic brown rice penne or rigatoni pasta
(One handful of dry pasta for each serving, plus 1 more handful)
Pinch of Himalayan pink sea salt
Organic extra virgin olive oil

*Basic Red Sauce, recipe on pg. 70*

Bring a large pot of water to a boil then add pasta and return to boil. Add a pinch of sea salt and cook pasta until el danté – do not overcook. Drain pasta. Pour a few drops of olive oil into the pot and return the pasta. Pour basic red sauce over pasta – enough to cover and mix through, adding more sauce if desired. Serve in individual pasta bowls and garnish with a piece of fresh basil if desired.

Optional: substitute rice pasta for any type of gluten-free pasta.
Optional: grate some fresh pecorino romano or parmesan cheese, or, dairy-free cheese substitute or nutritional yeast, if preferred.

*Be sure to check the beginning of the book in the TIPS section for many helpful hints, alternatives, substitutes or suggestions that could save time and energy!*

# Steamed Tilapia with Tamari Soy Sauce

Frozen tilapia fillets
1 tbsp. organic tamari soy sauce for each fillet

Place each fillet in foil, pour tamari soy sauce on top and wrap. Put into shallow baking dish or pan and bake at 375° for approx 20 minutes (cooking time will vary depending on size of fillets). For fresh fillets cook approx 6–8 minutes. Do not overcook.

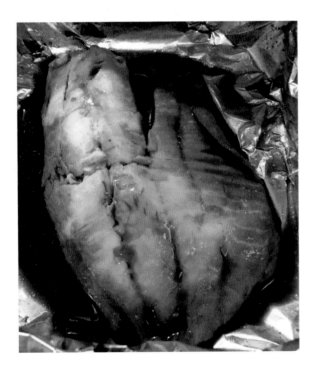

*Be sure to check the beginning of the book in the TIPS section for many helpful hints, alternatives, substitutes or suggestions that could save time and energy!*

# Stuffed Rolled Turkey Cutlet

2 organic turkey cutlets, tenderized
1 cup organic kale or swiss chard, chopped
3/4 cup crumbled goat feta cheese or dairy-free cheese substitute
1 tsp. organic garlic, chopped

Wash cutlets, tenderize with a mallet or tenderizing tool and place on a flat surface. Wash kale. Spread garlic over cutlets, cover with chopped kale or swiss chard, and sprinkle the crumbled goat feta or dairy-free cheese substitute all over. Roll up and tuck in each end. Secure with food ties or poultry string. Bake in preheated oven at 350° for 25–30 minutes.

*Be sure to check the beginning of the book in the TIPS section for many helpful hints, alternatives, substitutes or suggestions that could save time and energy!*

# Turkey Cacciatore

1 lb. organic turkey, ground or chunks of breast meat
1–2 tsp. organic extra virgin olive oil, grapeseed oil or avocado oil

*Basic Red Sauce, recipe on page 70*

1/2 cup organic red wine (for flavour)
1 med organic red onion, chopped
2-3 leaves of kale, chopped with stem removed
1 organic red pepper, chopped
2 stalks organic celery, chopped

Start with heating the Basic red sauce in large pot. Wash vegetables. In a med size frying pan, add 1 tsp. olive oil and heat; add chopped onion, peppers, celery and sauté for about 5 minutes. Add chopped kale and continue to cook for a few more minutes until leaves are tender. Remove and add to the basic red sauce. In frying pan add 1 tsp. olive oil and heat; add ground turkey and cook over med heat until meat starts to brown and there is no more pink. Remove and add to the sauce, simmering covered for 45 minutes. Add the red wine and continue to simmer for 15 more minutes. Serve with your favorite noodles; I like brown rice penne.

Optional: substitute turkey for chicken.

*Be sure to check the beginning of the book in the TIPS section for many helpful hints, alternatives, substitutes or suggestions that could save time and energy!*

# Turkey (or Chicken) Chili

5 cups organic roma tomatoes, chopped
1 pkg. ground organic turkey, or chicken
1 can organic chick peas, drained and rinsed
1 can organic black beans, drained and rinsed
1 cup organic broccoli, chopped
4 stalks organic celery, chopped
2 medium organic red onions, chopped
2 cloves organic garlic, chopped
1/2 cup hot chile peppers, chopped fine
1 tbsp. organic extra virgin olive oil, grapeseed oil or avocado oil
1/2 tsp. Himalayan pink sea salt

Wash vegetables. Brown the ground poultry in a large skillet
in a few drops of olive oil. Add the onion and cook on med for
about 10 minutes; may need to add a bit more olive oil. Add the
tomatoes, beans, garlic and chili peppers. Cook for 20–30 minutes
on med-low, add the celery and broccoli and reduce to simmer
for another 5–10 minutes enough to heat through but keeping the
celery crunchy.

*Be sure to check the beginning of the book in the TIPS section for many helpful
hints, alternatives, substitutes or suggestions that could save time and energy!*

## Chicken with Vegetables and Almonds

2 cups boneless skinless organic chicken cut into strips
1 cup organic broccoli, cut
1 cup organic celery, cut into large pieces
1 cup organic asparagus
2 tsp. organic extra virgin olive oil, grapeseed oil or avocado oil
2 tsp. organic tamari soy sauce
1/4 tsp. cayenne pepper
1/3 cup almonds glazed with cane sugar
Or 2 tsp. honey – optional

Wash all vegetables. Heat the pan with oil and add the chicken strips. Cook approx 5 minutes turning frequently to cook all sides. Add vegetables, cover and continue cooking on med heat for 5-7 minutes, stirring often. Remove lid, sprinkle the cayenne and add the soy sauce. Stir, reduce heat and cook down to reduce any excess liquid. Add glazed almonds (or almonds and honey) and stir through until mixed and heated. Serve with brown rice or quinoa.

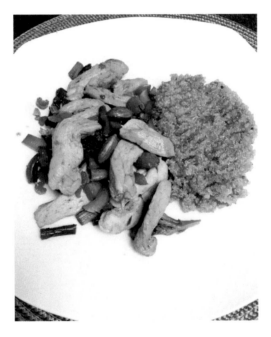

*Be sure to check the beginning of the book in the TIPS section for many helpful hints, alternatives, substitutes or suggestions that could save time and energy!*

# SWEETS AND TREATS

# Almond Macaroons

1 cup whole raw almonds
1/4 cup quinoa flour
3 whole egg whites (1/2 cup egg whites only)
2/3 cup sucanat (organic raw cane sugar)
1 tbsp. organic vanilla extract
1/2 tsp. ground organic cinnamon
1/2 tsp. Himalayan sea salt

Preheat oven to 325°. Place the almonds in a food processor or chopper and process until they resemble a course meal. Beat the egg whites until quite stiff, and then beat in the sucanat, vanilla, cinnamon and salt. Add the flour to the ground almonds and gently fold into the other ingredients. Drop from teaspoon on a greased baking sheet. Bake for 15 minutes or until edges are golden. Remove carefully with a spatula to cool on a rack. The cookies will become crispy when cooled. Store in an airtight container.

*Be sure to check the beginning of the book in the TIPS section for many helpful hints, alternatives, substitutes or suggestions that could save time and energy!*

# Carob Cookies

3/4 cup coconut flour
1/2 cup chickpea flour
1/2 cup brown rice flour
1/2 ripe avocado
1/3 cup currants or raisins
1/3 cup carob chips
1 tsp. organic vanilla
2 tbsp. unsweetened carob powder
1/2 tsp. gluten-free baking soda
1/2 cup organic raw honey
2 tbsp. organic maple syrup

Preheat oven to 350° Mix all flour, carob powder and baking soda in a bowl. In another bowl, mash avocado, then mix in honey, maple syrup and vanilla with a hand blender on low until smooth. Add to dry ingredients and blend together on low speed until mixed. Stir in currants and carob chips with a fork. Form a heaping spoonful into a ball in your hand and drop onto a non-stick cookie sheet then flatten slightly with a fork. You can also line the cookie sheet with parchment paper. Bake for 13–15 minutes or until edges are browning, do not overcook. Let cool 10 mins before removing. Store in an airtight container when cooled. Makes approx. 24 cookies.

Optional: replace carob chips and powder with chocolate and cocoa powder, if preferred.

*Be sure to check the beginning of the book in the TIPS section for many helpful hints, alternatives, substitutes or suggestions that could save time and energy!*

# Avocado Chocolate Mousse

2 ripe avocados (med – large size)
2 tbsp. organic dark maple syrup
1/3 cup organic cocoa powder
2 tbsp. organic cold-pressed coconut oil
1 tsp. organic vanilla extract
2/3 cup organic unsweetened coconut milk

Put all ingredients in a Vitamix or high-power blender and pureé until a nice smooth consistency. Transfer to small serving bowls and decorate with a sprinkling of fine shredded coconut or shaved chocolate. Refrigerate for at least 1 hour before serving. Makes 4–6 servings.

Optional: substitute unsweetened coconut milk with unsweetened almond, cashew, rice or hemp milk, if desired.

Optional: for added protein, add 2 tbsp. organic, plant-based protein powder. May need to add a bit more milk if this is too thick.

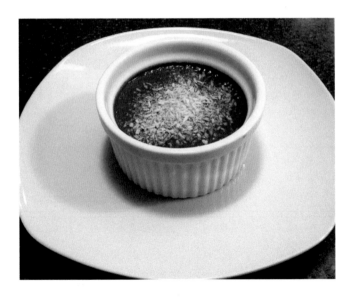

*Be sure to check the beginning of the book in the TIPS section for many helpful hints, alternatives, substitutes or suggestions that could save time and energy!*

# Chocolate Almond Cookies

3/4 cup raw almond butter (can use any nut or seed butter)
1/4 cup raw pumpkin butter (or adjust almond butter to 1 cup)
2 egg whites (1/3 cup egg whites only)
2 tbsp. unsweetened almond milk
2/3 cup organic raw cane sugar
2/3 cup quinoa flour
1 tsp. gluten-free baking soda
1/2 tsp. organic vanilla extract
3/4 cup organic diary-free dark unsweetened chocolate chips or chunks

Preheat oven to 350°. In a medium bowl, stir together the almond butter, pumpkin butter, egg whites almond milk and vanilla. Add the cane sugar and mix, then add the flour, baking soda and fold together until blended. Mix in the chocolate. Drop from teaspoon onto greased baking sheet (cookies will expand). Bake 10–12 minutes until the edges are browning. Let cool on a rack for approximately 30 minutes. Store in an airtight container.

*Be sure to check the beginning of the book in the TIPS section for many helpful hints, alternatives, substitutes or suggestions that could save time and energy!*

# Chocolatey Chia Pudding

1 1/2 cups organic unsweetened coconut milk
1/4 cup organic cocoa powder
1/3 cup chia seeds
1 tbsp. organic maple syrup
1 tsp. organic vanilla extract
1/4 tsp. Himalayan pink sea salt

Put all ingredients in a mason jar and stir to remove any lumps, then shake well to thoroughly mix. Let sit for 10 mins, shake again then sit for another 20 minutes before pouring into small individual serving dishes and put in the fridge for at least 4 hours to set. Makes 4–6 servings.

Optional: substitute unsweetened coconut milk with unsweetened almond, cashew, rice or hemp milk, if desired.

*Be sure to check the beginning of the book in the TIPS section for many helpful hints, alternatives, substitutes or suggestions that could save time and energy!*

# Coconut Sprouted Almond Cookies

1/2 cup ground sprouted almonds*
3/4 cup coconut flour
3-4 tbsp. coconut butter
2/3 cup organic raw honey
3 tbsp. egg whites
1/2 tsp. organic vanilla extract
1/3 cup organic diary-free dark unsweetened chocolate chips
1/2 tsp. gluten-free baking soda
Up to 1 tbsp. of water

Preheat oven to 350°. Line a baking sheet with parchment paper. In a large bowl mix together the coconut butter, honey, egg whites and vanilla. Add the flour, ground almonds and chocolate chips mixing until all combined. May need to add up to 1 tbsp. of water if too dry. Drop from teaspoon onto baking sheet, leaving space to expand. Bake for 15 minutes or until browning. Remove from oven and leave on baking sheet for 15 minutes before removing to cooling rack. Store in an airtight container.

*Sprouted almonds – Soak raw almonds in water for 8 hours or overnight. Drain, rinse and drain again to remove as much water as possible. Store in a sealed container in the fridge for up to 7 days. The almonds don't actually grow sprouts however, are much more nutritious, provide more protein and easier to digest once soaked. The same is true with soaking all raw nuts before eating them.

*Be sure to check the beginning of the book in the TIPS section for many helpful hints, alternatives, substitutes or suggestions that could save time and energy!*

# Coconut Vanilla Chia Pudding

1 1/2 cups organic unsweetened coconut milk
1/4 cup organic unsweetened finely shredded coconut
1/4 cup chia seeds
1 tbsp. organic maple syrup
1 tsp. organic vanilla extract
1/4 tsp. Himalayan pink sea salt

Put all ingredients in a mason jar and stir to remove any lumps, then shake well to thoroughly mix. Let sit for 10 mins, shake again then sit for another 20 minutes before pouring into small individual serving dishes and put in the fridge for at least 4 hours to set. Makes 4–6 servings.

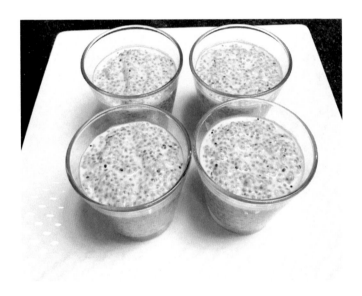

*Be sure to check the beginning of the book in the TIPS section for many helpful hints, alternatives, substitutes or suggestions that could save time and energy!*

# Coconut Nog Latte

Organic espresso beans (regular or decaffeinated)
1/2 cup plain organic coconut milk
1/4 cup coconut nog
Organic cinnamon

Make espresso (or coffee) per the instructions for your equipment. Mix coconut milk and coconut nog together and heat gently but don't burn. Whip with milk frother or steam in espresso machine to create a thick foam. Pour over espresso and spoon foam on top. Sprinkle with cinnamon, if desired.

*Be sure to check the beginning of the book in the TIPS section for many helpful hints, alternatives, substitutes or suggestions that could save time and energy!*

# Crispy Nut Butter Cookies

1/2 cup pure organic honey
1/2 cup ripe avocado (or banana)
1/3 cup pure organic maple syrup
1/2 cup organic nut or seed butter (almond, pumpkin, cashew)
1/2 tsp. organic vanilla extract
1 cup brown rice flour
1 cup chickpea flour
1 cup brown rice flakes
1 tsp. gluten-free baking soda
Pinch of Himalayan pink sea salt
1/2 cup walnuts, chopped

Preheat oven to 350°. Beat honey, maple syrup, avocado, nut
butter and vanilla in med bowl until creamy. Mix flour, half of the
flakes, baking soda and salt together in a small bowl. Mix in with
other ingredients, add nuts and stir until well blended. Drop from
rounded teaspoon to cookie sheet lined with parchment paper.
Spread some flakes on a small plate, dip fork in flakes and then
press to slightly flatten cookies before baking. Bake for 13–15
minutes. Cool 3 minutes before removing.

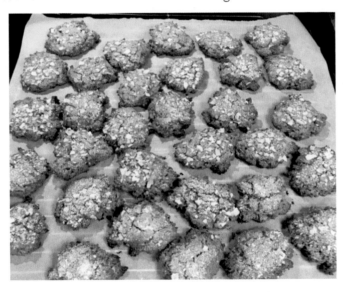

*Be sure to check the beginning of the book in the TIPS section for many helpful
hints, alternatives, substitutes or suggestions that could save time and energy!*

# Gluten and Dairy-free Muffins

1 cup organic apple sauce
1/3 cup organic extra virgin olive oil or avocado oil
1/2 cup organic honey
3/4 cup chickpea flour
1 cup brown rice flour
1 egg equivalent*
1 tsp. organic vanilla
1 tsp. gluten-free baking soda
1 tsp. gluten-free baking powder
1 tsp. Himalayan pink sea salt
1/2 cup walnuts, chopped fine
1cup frozen berries (raspberries, blueberries or cranberries)

*1 egg equivalent: 1 tbsp. ground flax seed mixed with 3 tbsp. of water and let stand for 2 minutes then mix together*

Preheat oven to 325°. Mix applesauce, oil, honey and sea salt. Add egg substitute, vanilla and beat well. Add in flour, baking soda, baking powder and mix until blended. Add nuts and berries and gently fold in. Fill lined muffin tins 3/4 full and bake for 20–25 minutes. Test center clean with a toothpick.

*Be sure to check the beginning of the book in the TIPS section for many helpful hints, alternatives, substitutes or suggestions that could save time and energy!*

# Raw Organic Chocolate

1 cup organic cold-pressed coconut oil
1/2 cup organic maple syrup
1/4 cup raw organic unpasteurized honey
1 tsp. organic vanilla extract
1 1/4 cup organic cocoa powder
Shredded unsweetened organic coconut for decorating

Put a medium sized bowl over a pot of hot water. Don't let the bowl touch the water so not much water is needed. Add the coconut oil and the honey to the bowl and melt together. Remove from heat, add the maple syrup, vanilla and cocoa powder, whisking together until completely blended, working quickly before it starts to set. Pour onto a cookie sheet lined with parchment paper and smooth it out with a spatula for even thickness. Decorate with a light dusting of cocoa powder and/or fine shredded coconut and place in freezer for approximately 15 minutes to set, then remove and cut into bite sized pieces. Store in a sealed container in the fridge or freezer.

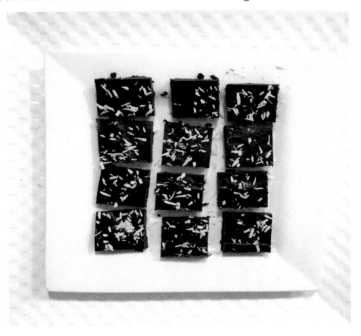

*Be sure to check the beginning of the book in the TIPS section for many helpful hints, alternatives, substitutes or suggestions that could save time and energy!*

# Raw Almond Coconut Truffles

2 cups organic unsweetened coconut, shredded or grated
1 cup raw (soaked) almonds, chopped fine (soak in filtered water for 8 hours, drain and rinse)
1 cup organic cold-pressed coconut oil
3/4 cup organic cocoa powder
1/2 cup organic maple syrup
1/4 cup chia seeds
2 tbsp. ground flax seed
1 tsp. organic cinnamon

Chop almonds in a food processor. Whisk coconut oil in a large bowl until smooth and soft. Add all ingredients and combine until thoroughly mixed. Place in the fridge for about 15 minutes to allow coconut oil to harden a bit. Remove and begin to form small balls about 1/2" in size and place on a cookie sheet covered in parchment paper. Return to the fridge to completely set for about an hour and then decorate with a light dusting of cocoa powder or roll in fine shredded coconut and then store in an airtight container. They can be kept in the fridge or freezer until serving.

*Be sure to check the beginning of the book in the TIPS section for many helpful hints, alternatives, substitutes or suggestions that could save time and energy!*

# Gluten-free Organic Brownies

2 eggs or egg replacement
1 tsp. organic vanilla
1/4 tsp. Himalayan pink sea salt
3/4 cup coconut flour
1/2 cup coconut or cane sugar
1/4 cup organic dark maple syrup
2 tbsp. coconut or almond milk

1/2 cup melted coconut oil
3/4 tsp. baking powder
1/2 cup raw cocoa powder
1/4 cup almond flour

1/2 cup non-dairy semi-sweet chocolate chips or walnuts (or 1/4 cup of each)
3/4 cup non-diary semi-sweet chocolate chips for the topping
1 tbsp. organic unsweetened coconut, shredded Or finely chopped walnuts

Preheat oven to 350°. Lightly grease an 8 x 8 baking dish with coconut oil. I like to use a zip lock bag as a glove and grab some coconut oil to rub in the baking dish. It is easy to spread and doesn't get your hand greasy. Line the baking dish with parchment paper tight to the sides.

In a large bowl add the melted coconut oil, coconut sugar, maple syrup and vanilla and whisk to blend. Add the eggs and whisk in, add baking powder, sea salt, cocoa powder and whisk all together. Add the coconut flour and almond flour and fold in with a spatula just to blend. Add 2–3 tbsp. of coconut or almond milk if too dry. Add the chocolate chips (and walnuts) and gently fold in.

Spread the batter in the lined baking dish and even out to the corners. Bake for 20–23 minutes until the edges are dry and the center is not wet on a toothpick.

Remove from oven and spread 1 cup of additional chocolate chips and let it sit for 5–10 minutes to melt. Once all melted, spread evenly with the back of a spoon and decorate with a sprinkling of shredded coconut or chopped nuts.

Let cool 45 mins before cutting in squares. Store in an airtight container in the fridge or freezer.

*Be sure to check the beginning of the book in the TIPS section for many helpful hints, alternatives, substitutes or suggestions that could save time and energy!*

# Index

# Index

# Index

# Index

Made in the USA
Middletown, DE
27 November 2023

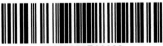

43627375R00082